Sports Injuries of the
Ankle and Foot

Springer
New York
Berlin
Heidelberg
Barcelona
Budapest
Hong Kong
London
Milan
Paris
Santa Clara
Singapore
Tokyo

Richard A. Marder   George J. Lian
University of California Davis School of Medicine

Sports Injuries of the Ankle and Foot

Line Illustrations by Justin Green

With 151 Figures, 16 in Color

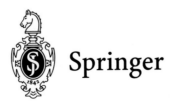

Springer

Richard A. Marder, MD
Associate Professor
University of California Davis
School of Medicine
Chief, Sports Medicine Service
1631 Stockton Boulevard, Suite 120
Sacramento, CA 95816, USA

George J. Lian, MD
Assistant Clinical Professor
University of California Davis
School of Medicine
Department of Orthopaedic Surgery
1201 Alhambra Boulevard, Suite 310
Sacramento, CA 95816, USA

Library of Congress Cataloging in Publication Data

RD 563
. M 359
1997

Marder, Richard A.
    Sports injuries of the ankle and foot / Richard A.
Marder, George J. Lian
      p. cm.
    Includes bibliographical references and index.
    ISBN 0-387-94687-X (alk. paper)
    1. Foot—Wounds and injuries. 2. Ankle—Wounds and injuries.
3. Sports injuries. I. Marder, Richard A. II. Title.
    [DNLM: 1. Ankle Injuries—therapy. 2. Foot Injuries—therapy.
3. Sports Medicine. WE 880 L693s 1996]
RD563.L52 1996
617.5'85044—dc20
DNLM/DLC
for Library of Congress   96-7605

Printed on acid-free paper.

Production coordinated by Chernow Editorial Services, Inc. and managed by Terry
Kornak; manufacturing supervised by Jeffrey Taub.
Typeset by TechType, Inc., Ramsey, NJ.
Printed and bound by Maple-Vail Book Manufacturing Group, York, PA.
Printed in the United States of America.

9 8 7 6 5 4 3 2 1

ISBN 0-387-94687-X Springer-Verlag New York Berlin Heidelberg SPIN 10524824

To our families, for their love and support

Preface

The ultimate aim of a medical textbook is to benefit patients. In this instance it is directed at the treatment of ankle and foot injuries and disorders in both recreational and high performance athletes. Our goal is not to proselytize but to present cogent, practical information in the framework of a readable text. The book is not encyclopedic in its contents; instead, we focus on the treatment of common injuries and conditions, both operative and nonoperative treatment, as well as the all important rehabilitation phase, which facilitates the athlete's return to sport. A chapter on taping, orthotics, and braces has been included to enhance the understanding of their use for treatment and injury prevention.

We have organized the book into sections based on anatomic region where appropriate and by type of injury otherwise. The differential diagnosis of presenting symptoms and signs is discussed, leading to some repetition of material. The book is intended to reflect our philosophies regarding treatment. Despite myriad treatment possibilities, we have chosen only those primary and alternative methods with which we have had significant experience. The inspiration for this book comes from patients, therapists, instructors, and colleagues who have educated and stimulated us to continue to improve our efforts to help patients. We hope this reference will be useful to other physicians and ultimately their patients.

Contents

Introduction: Special Considerations in the Athlete

Injuries of the foot and ankle occur frequently in sports. Moreover, a significant number of atraumatic conditions, not manifest during normal activity, can become symptomatic owing to the increased demands of sport. Although certain of these injuries and conditions resolve spontaneously, a significant number require formal treatment.

The fundamental tenet of orthopaedic treatment is to restore function whenever possible. Maximizing functional recovery is of utmost importance in the athlete. Whereas postinjury functional deficits may not be noticeable in the less active individual, even slight functional loss in an athlete can impair performance or potentially prevent participation. As there are currently no standards by which to predict return to sport after an injury, the treating physician should strive to achieve full anatomic and functional restoration of the foot and ankle. In most cases treatment of the injured athlete starts with several advantages that help to promote an optimal outcome. Despite injury, the athlete usually has a high level of fitness, which is conducive to prompt, uneventful healing. The motivation of the athlete to return to sport usually ensures compliance with a rigorous rehabilitation regimen necessary to promote maximal soft tissue recovery. The importance of dedicated trainers and therapists, who assist the athlete in his or her endeavors, usually on a daily basis, cannot be overemphasized.

Given the large numbers of potential injuries with time lost from sport, prevention is paramount. For the foot and ankle, shoewear, orthotics, braces, and taping are frequently utilized. Use of these devices and methods varies considerably, based on the experiences of the individual player, trainer, and physician. Scientific studies have been undertaken to demonstrate their efficacy. It is helpful for the physician treating athletes with ankle and foot disorders to have a working knowledge of such protective equipment.

When treating the athlete the physician must be aware that the recommended treatment may not be accepted by the patient. For instance, although rest from activity may be indicated for an overuse injury, the serious athlete in the middle of the season may not be willing to stop unless forced to do so by the injury. Instead, simultaneous treatment and activity modification may have to be utilized in which the athlete may reduce the intensity of practice and the number of minutes played, as well as forego "back to back" games, for example. Of more potential seriousness is the timing of surgery for chronic or even acute conditions in the high performance athlete. Whereas immediate surgery may be the optimal treatment, the athlete may choose to continue playing for the season, deferring surgery until afterward. The physician must discuss, in detail, the consequences of postponing treatment (e.g., the development of degenerative arthritis, which could impair future ability to play and interfere with even routine activities). Such discussion should be well documented in the medical record and, if the player concurs, discussed with his or her family, coach, and trainer.

Of added importance for treatment of the high performance athlete (high school, college, professional) is the need to formulate a detailed treatment plan at the outset that covers not only the proposed surgical procedure, for instance, but potential complications and contingency plans, formal rehabilitation, and finally transition to functional exercises and activities in preparation for return to sport. Inclusion of family, coaches, trainers, management, and agents in the initial discussion of the injury and treatment plan, per the approval of the player, can greatly improve the chances for a successful outcome.

Notwithstanding the ever-increasing numbers of high performance athletes, most patients with foot and ankle injuries are recreational-level participants. For these patients limited time for rehabilitation exercises and, in many instances, restricted access to formal therapy may require some modification of treatment programs customarily utilized for the high performance athlete. Especially for the recreational athlete, who may be knowledgeable about injuries in famous professional and amateur athletes, it is helpful for the treating physician to discuss with the patient that no two injuries are alike and that different outcomes may result, even with the same treatment from the same physician.

Finally and most importantly, the physician must remember that the athlete, regardless of stature and fame, is susceptible to frustration, anger, and despair when dealing with an injury that does not heal quickly and uneventfully. Frequent communication, appropriate compassion, and second opinions are helpful for maintaining a successful doctor–patient relationship during this time.

1
Ankle

Ligament Injuries

Lateral Ankle Ligament

Tears of the lateral ankle ligaments are among the most common sports injuries (Jackson et al., 1974). The spectrum of injury ranges from mild sprains, after which an athlete might return to activity the same day, to frank rupture of one or more ligaments, which can cause considerable lost time from sport and persistent symptoms. Furthermore, chronic lateral instability occurs in nearly 20% of patients (Boruta et al., 1990; Freeman, 1965; Freeman et al., 1965; Kannus and Renstrom, 1991; Rijke et al., 1988).

Because of these potential postinjury sequelae, it is incumbent on physicians involved in the treatment of athletes to have knowledge of injury prevention as well as of effective therapeutic regimens. Of additional significance is that a number of conditions, including peroneal tendon dislocation, midfoot and subtalar injuries, and osteochondral lesions, can mimic lateral ankle ligament injury.

Biomechanics and Injury

The lateral ankle capsule is reinforced by three ligaments: the anterior and posterior talofibular ligaments and the calcaneofibular ligament. Clinically, the anterior talofibular and calcaneofibular ligaments are the most important, as these ligaments function in a reciprocal manner to resist inversion forces applied to the ankle. The anterior talofibular ligament develops increasing strain as the ankle is moved from dorsiflexion to plantarflexion, and the calcaneofibular ligament develops its highest strain in dorsiflexion (Colville et al., 1992; Renstrom et al., 1988). The calcaneofibular ligament, because of its anatomic orientation, also stabilizes the subtalar joint (Heilman et al., 1990; Laurin et al., 1968).

The lateral ankle ligaments are injured by inversion forces being applied to the plantarflexed ankle during loading or unloading of the ankle. Injury affects the anterior talofibular ligament first, followed by the calcaneofibular ligament (Anderson et al., 1952; Brostrom, 1964; Dias, 1979; Rasmussen, 1985). With extreme forces, the posterior talofibular ligament can rupture, causing dislocation of the talus. Whereas isolated injury of the anterior talofibular ligament is common, isolated rupture of the calcaneofibular ligament is clinically unlikely (Brostrom, 1964; Rasmussen, 1985).

Clinical Presentation

From the history one can determine the level of athletic performance, ascertain any previous ankle injury, reconstruct the mechanism of injury, elicit the occurrence of a pop or tearing sensation, note whether the individual continued playing or is unable to bear weight, and establish the onset and location of swelling. Obviously, the ability to continue playing and the presence of minimal swelling suggest a mild or moderate injury, whereas rapid swelling, inability to bear weight, and continued pain portend more severe injury.

A comprehensive examination of the ankle and foot is important to avoid missing associated and adjacent injuries. Inspection, palpation, neuromuscular tests, and laxity tests comprise the foundation of the physical examination.

Swelling always occurs with a complete ligament tear, and ecchymosis develops in approximately one-half of patients (Brostrom, 1964). If the patient is examined within a few hours of injury, swelling is seen to be localized to the inframalleolar region and can be differentiated from the supramalleolar swelling seen with syndesmosis injury or fibular fracture, and the more distal swelling over the sinus tarsi and midfoot due to subtalar or midfoot sprains and fracture of the anterior process of the calcaneus.

The malleoli, medial and lateral ankle capsule and ligaments, anterior and posterior margins of the tibiotalar joint, tibiofibular syndesmosis and the entire length of the fibula, peroneal and Achilles tendons, and the sinus tarsi must be palpated. Tenderness of an individual ligament is suggestive of, but not specific for, injury of that ligament.

The active range of ankle motion is measured; passive motion is painful and does not aid in diagnosis. Evaluation of peroneal muscle function is important. Active dorsiflexion and eversion may demonstrate dislocation of the peroneal tendons. Test the integrity of the peroneal tendons by having the patient evert the foot against resistance. Palpate the pedal pulses and complete the sensory and motor examination of the foot and ankle. Traction injuries of the posterior tibial and peroneal nerves and peroneal compartment syndromes have been described following severe ankle ligament injuries (Nitz et al., 1985; Singer and Jones, 1986).

Laxity Tests

The lateral ligaments are evaluated by the anterior drawer and talar tilt tests. The ante-

rior drawer test measures anterior displacement of the talus in relation to the tibia (Anderson et al., 1952; Dehne, 1934). The primary restraint to this test is the anterior talofibular ligament. Maximum talar translation occurs with testing in 10 degrees of plantarflexion (Grace, 1984). Injury of the calcaneofibular ligament does not affect the anterior drawer test (Larsen, 1985).

Talar instability is also assessed by the talar tilt test. This test is useful for evaluating combined injuries of the anterior talofibular and calcaneofibular ligaments. The initial restraint to talar tilt in plantarflexion is the anterior talofibular ligament. The secondary restraint is the calcaneofibular ligament. Rupture of the anterior talofibular ligament produces only a small increase in talar tilt, but rupture of the calcaneofibular ligament as well further increases the tilt.

The anterior drawer test is performed with the patient supine or sitting. In the sitting position, allow the knee to flex over the edge of the table or bench with the ankle in 10 degrees of plantarflexion. Stabilize the anterior aspect of the distal leg with one hand and apply an anterior force to the heel with the other, attempting to subluxate the talus anteriorly. An alternative method is the modified anterior drawer test performed with the patient supine (Nyska et al., 1992). The knee is flexed to approximately 120 degrees, and the foot is fixed to the table or ground by one hand of the examiner, maintaining the ankle in 10 degrees of plantarflexion. The examiner's other hand applies a posteriorly directed force to the anterior distal leg, attempting to translate the tibia posteriorly. Neither test is usually painful, and each can be performed in the presence of established swelling. Comparison with the other ankle allows determination of a normal or abnormal test. If the test demonstrates an abnormal increase, stress radiographs are obtained to allow quantification of laxity.

The talar tilt test is performed with the knee flexed over the side of the table or bench and the ankle in 10 degrees of plantarflexion. While the distal leg is stabilized by one hand of the examiner proximal to the medial malleolus, the other hand applies an inversion force to the hindfoot. The thumb of the hand applying the inversion force can be used to determine if tilting is occurring at the tibiotalar joint. An overall increase in inversion motion compared with the normal ankle indicates subtalar instability alone or combined with lateral ankle instability. This situation is more likely to be encountered in the patient being evaluated for symptoms suggesting recurrent instability. Unless gross ankle instability exists or the ankle is examined immediately or with anesthesia, the talar tilt test is unlikely to be markedly positive.

Because of the difficulty of accurately measuring joint laxity in the patient with an acute injury, stress radiographs are sometimes useful in patients whose clinical examination suggests abnormal laxity. They may also be helpful in patients with pain, swelling, or muscle spasm to a degree that prevents satisfactory assessment.

Radiography

Anteroposterior (AP), mortise, and lateral radiographs of the ankle are obtained routinely after suspected injury of the lateral ligaments. Associated osteochondral injuries, avulsions from the tip of the fibula, unsuspected disruption of the mortise, and malleolar fractures may be evident. In addition, if swelling and tenderness appear distal to the lateral malleolus along the lateral foot, a medial oblique and an AP view of the foot may demonstrate an anterior process fracture of the calcaneus or fracture of the base of the fifth metatarsal.

If the anterior drawer test is negative (3 mm or less side to side difference) and the talar tilt test is negative, stress radiographs are unnecessary. If desired, document the degree of laxity, obtaining both anterior drawer and talar tilt stress radiographs. The anterior drawer test is performed with the ankle in 10 degrees of plantarflexion. The talar tilt test is performed by having the patient seated with the hip and knee both flexed and the leg internally rotated 15 degrees. If necessary, inject 15 ml of 1% lidocaine into the ankle for pain relief. Obtain similar stress radiographs of the normal ankle.

The amount of anterior talar translation is measured as the distance from a constant point on the posterior aspect of the talus to the posterior lip of the tibia. A more than 3 mm side-to-side difference indicates a complete tear of the anterior talofibular ligament (Fig. 1.1) If there is 10 degrees or more side-to-side difference on the talar tilt test, both the anterior talofibular and calcaneofibular ligaments are ruptured (Fig. 1.2).

Ankle Arthrography and Magnetic Resonance Imagining

In the past, ankle arthrography and peroneal tenography were utilized to diagnose lateral ankle ligament tears (Fig. 1.3). Despite the ability of these contrast studies to demonstrate the anatomic extent of the injury, their use has declined because so few acute lateral ligament injuries are treated by early surgery. Similarly, magnetic resonance imaging (MRI) can demonstrate the anatomy of the injury. Because of its costliness, MRI is best reserved for investigating suspected osteochondral lesions of the talus and peroneal tendon tears.

Diagnosis

The mechanism of the injury, localized swelling, and tenderness suggest the diagnosis. In

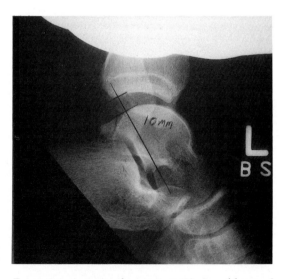

FIGURE 1.1. Anterior drawer test: 10 mm of forward displacement of the talus from the posterior lip of the tibia.

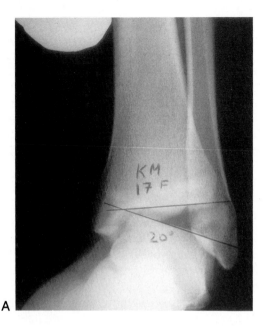

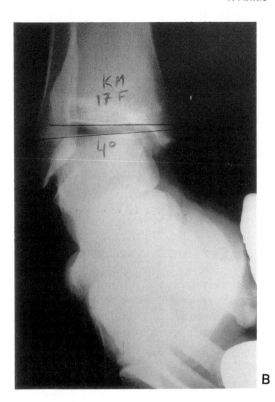

FIGURE 1.2A,B. Talar tilt test: 16 degrees side-to-side difference.

the absence of a demonstrable increase in laxity by clinical and radiographic stress tests, exclusion of other diagnoses is necessary. The differential diagnosis includes peroneal tendon subluxation, osteochondral lesions of the talus, and injuries of the subtalar and midfoot.

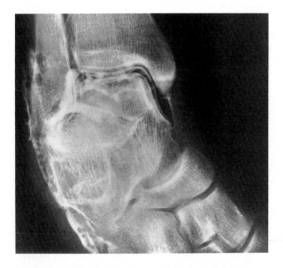

FIGURE 1.3. Peroneal tenography with dye extravasating into the ankle joint, indicating capsular rupture.

Classification

Ligament injuries are typically graded as first, second, or third degree, depending on their severity. Other classification schemes have been used for lateral ankle injuries, however, because these injuries are complex. Previously, when surgical repair was frequently performed for acute injuries, the concept of single and double ligament injuries became popular (Black et al., 1978). From a functional viewpoint, lateral ankle injuries are often classified as stable or unstable (Singer and Jones, 1986).

A classification scheme is valuable only if it assists in the formulation of treatment, helps to predict outcome, or facilitates comparison of treatment plans. Previously, classification has attempted to identify the patient who should have surgical repair of acutely torn lateral ankle ligaments. At present, because nonoperative treatment has become the norm for the treatment of most acute injuries, we have not chosen to utilize any specific classification. Rather, as a basis for ongoing study of residual symptoms after acute injuries, we attempt to define as precisely as possible the amount of initial laxity, using clinical and radiographic stress tests (anterior drawer and talar tilt).

Prevention

A number of preventive measures are routinely employed (i.e., taping and braces). As measured by biomechanical tests, taping can reduce inversion of the foot, but the effect is gradually lost during exercise (Greene and Hillman, 1990). Semirigid braces (Fig. 1.4) have been shown to decrease inversion and reduce the incidence of lateral ankle sprains. Despite the mechanical support offered by taping and orthoses, proprioceptive stimulation may in fact be a more significant effect (Lofvenberg et al., 1995). High-top shoes have been shown to reduce the amount of inversion of the plantarflexed ankle (Ottaviani et al., 1995). A prospective, randomized clinical study, however, has demonstrated no

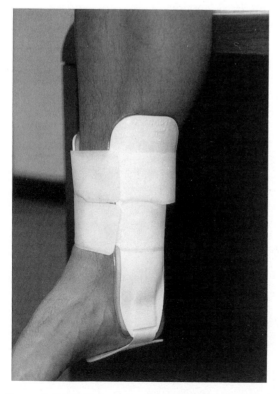

FIGURE 1.4. Rigid stirrup orthosis for ankle support.

measurable reduction in the ankle sprain injury rate from use of a high-top shoe compared to a low-top shoe (Barrett et al., 1993).

Treatment of Acute Injuries

Although the goal of treatment for all patients is to achieve a painless, stable ankle with normal motion, for athletes minimizing the time to return to activity is usually an added consideration. Thus if we assume equal outcomes from different treatments, the ideal treatment would be the one that resulted in the quickest return to sport. There are two major categories of treatment: operative and nonoperative.

Historically, operative repairs of significant ligament injuries have been standard treatment. Controlled studies, however, have shown no differences between the results of surgery and nonoperative methods (Evans et a., 1984; Freeman, 1965; Kannus and Renstrom, 1991; Moller-Larsen et al., 1988). In fact, both groups have approximately the same number of patients who subsequently experience chronic instability. Given these facts, together with the knowledge that surgical repair usually means the end of the season for the athlete, we reserve surgical treatment for the rare bony avulsion injury (Fig. 1.5) and the acute injuries that occur in the athlete with a history of severe, recurrent lateral ligament injury.

Nonoperative methods consist of immobilization and functional regimens emphasizing early joint mobilization with graduated rehabilitation. Provided there is access to supervised therapeutic modalities on a daily or, less desirable, an every other day basis, we prefer to institute a functional program for the athlete, regardless of the degree of documented laxity. Otherwise, initial splinting and cast immobilization are utilized for a maximum of 3 weeks, followed by a 1 to 2-week period of supervised rehabilitation.

Functional Rehabilitation

The mnemonic RICE (rest, ice, compression, elevation) is well known. Treatment starts once the severity of injury determines that

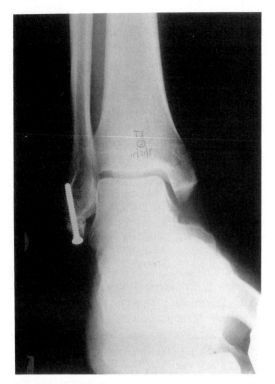

pression is applied in the treatment room (Fig. 1.6). Otherwise, the ankle and foot are immersed in an ice-water whirlpool or bucket for up to 25 minutes. Following this phase, a uniform compression bandage is applied that consists of a felt pad placed around the lateral malleolus in a "horseshoe" and secured with cast padding and tape. If ambulation is painful or the player is observed to limp, crutches are utilized. The athlete is instructed to keep the lower extremity elevated as much as possible for the first few days. Mild analgesics or nonsteroidal antiinflammatory drugs (NSAIDs) are often useful.

Usually the severity of the injury—as defined by pain, swelling, limited ability to bear weight unsupported, and loss of ankle motion—is evident on reinspection 24 to 48 hours postinjury. As Garrick (1981) noted, the resolution of swelling and pain are important milestones that determine the progression of functional rehabilitation.

FIGURE 1.5. Fixation of an avulsion fracture of the tip of the lateral malleolus, which contains the attachments of the anterior talofibular and calcaneofibular ligaments.

Therapy Schedule

The sequence of the treatment regimen is a modified version of the one suggested by Garrick (1981).

the player is unable to continue playing. If available, a commercial ankle boot that delivers intermittent cold and mechanical com-

Days 2 to 7

Cryotherapy and compression are continued. An inferential unit may help relieve pain.

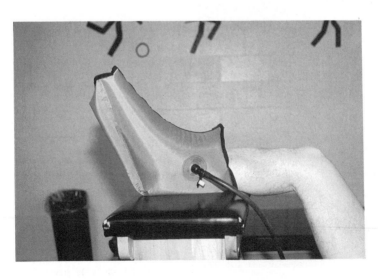

FIGURE 1.6. Cryo-compression boot.

Ankle motion, both active and passive, are started. Motion can be performed in a cold whirlpool both to take advantage of its anesthetic effect. Theraband, surgical tubing, and similar cord-like devices are useful for starting active resistive exercises in the pain-free range. Although plantarflexion and inversion are performed, emphasis is on eversion and dorsiflexion motions. The stationary bicycle is useful for motion as well. Proprioceptive exercises using a tilt board (Fig. 1.7), and manual resistive ankle exercises can usually be started at the end of this period.

Days 5 to 10

Ice and compression are no longer usually needed; and if desired, heat can be instituted. Most patients are ambulating pain-free. Isotonic exercises are instituted. Use of a stationary bike with tension is encouraged. Fast walking is started on a treadmill. Treadmill speed toward running follows when ankle

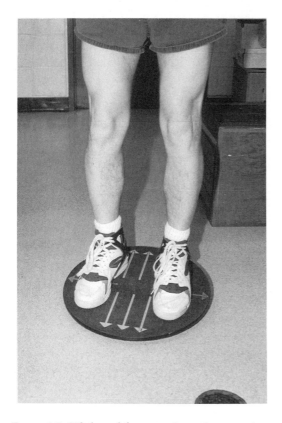

FIGURE 1.7. Tilt board for proprioceptive exercises.

motion and strength are near normal. Strength can be assessed by manual resistance, isotonic, or isokinetic testing. Taping or an ankle orthosis should be used during this phase.

Days 7 to 21

Functional exercises (e.g., figure-of-eights, backward running, pivoting) are allowed with the patient using ankle support. Progression to sport specific drills are next, followed by return to activity. The athlete continues to use an ankle support for the remainder of the season.

Postinjury Complications

A number of patients experience residual symptoms after a routine inversion injury. Postsprain complications include ankle pain secondary to osteochondral lesions, ossicles, or the development of a soft tissue impingement syndrome at the anterolateral corner of the tibiotalar articulation (Basett et al., 1990; Ferkel et al., 1991; Meislen et al., 1993; Taga et al., 1993). As previously noted, the most frequent problem is chronic instability.

Chronic Lateral Ankle Instability

Assessment

After one or more inversion injuries, the patient may note continuing pain, swelling, giving-way, or functional instability associated with pivoting and twisting on the ankle and foot. Physical examination can demonstrate peroneal weakness and calf atrophy, tenderness to palpation over the lateral ligaments with chronic soft tissue swelling in the inframalleolar region, and most significantly abnormal laxity during the anterior drawer and talar tilt tests. Routine radiographs may demonstrate ossicles about the tip of the lateral malleolus. The key to establishing the diagnosis is the demonstration of abnormal laxity on stress radiographs as described previously.

In the presence of symptoms not substantiated by radiographically confirmed laxity, another diagnosis must be considered. Peroneal subluxation can be diagnosed by observing retromalleolar tenderness and crepitus, being able to displace the tendons on examination, or spontaneous subluxation of the tendons from the peroneal groove on active dorsiflexion and eversion of the foot and ankle. Subtalar instability, which can mimic or coexist with lateral ankle instability, should be suspected if total subtalar inversion exceeds that on the normal side. However, subtalar instability may go undetected unless stress radiographs are obtained or stress tomography of the subtalar joint is performed (Laurin et al., 1968). In the absence of mechanical instability, loose bodies or ossicles at the tip of the lateral malleolus can produce symptoms of instability. Functional instability, as popularized by Freeman et al. (1965), is thought to be due to loss of proprioception after lateral ligament injury and is ameliorated by the same nonoperative exercise programs as are utilized for mechanical instability.

Nonoperative Treatment

Most patients with symptomatic mechanical lateral instability of the ankle respond to a program of peroneal strengthening, proprioceptive training, and use of an ankle orthosis, brace, or taping, as described above. Tilt boards are especially helpful for reconditioning the ankle and lower leg, facilitating transition to sport.

Operative Treatment

There are two types of basic operative procedures: delayed repair of the torn ligaments and reconstruction (Brostrom, 1966; Chrisman and Snook, 1969; Colville and Grondel, 1995; Evans, 1953; Watson-Jones, 1955). Success rates are approximately 85% irrespective of procedure. In most instances, delayed primary repair of the anterior talofibular and calcaneofibular ligaments is possible and, as such, is the procedure of choice. Potential disadvantages of reconstructive procedures include limitation of ankle and subtalar motion due to the nonanatomic location of the tendon graft and local morbidity from graft harvest (Burks and Morgan, 1994; Colville et al., 1992). Indications for reconstruction as opposed to delayed primary re-

pair include severe lateral ankle instability of long duration, evidence of subtalar hypermobility, or failure of a previous reconstruction (Colville and Grondel, 1995).

Delayed Primary Repair

Surgical Technique. This technique is a modification of the one described by Brostrom (1966).

1. Administer a prophylactic antibiotic, usually cefazolin. Perform arthroscopy, if desired, as a significant number of patients have chondral lesions of the medial talar dome.
2. Place a bump underneath the ipsilateral hip of the supine patient to internally rotate the foot and ankle.
3. Under tourniquet control, incise the skin starting along the anterior border of the lateral malleolus 3 cm proximal to the tip, gently curving posteriorly and inferiorly to the visible and palpable peroneal tendons. Alternately, with the ankle in maximum equinus, place the skin incision immediately posterior to the prominence of the lateral malleolus, starting 3 cm proximal to the tip and following the peroneal tendons distally (Fig. 1.8). This incision

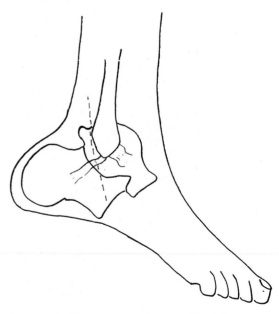

FIGURE 1.8. Skin incision for modified Brostrom procedure.

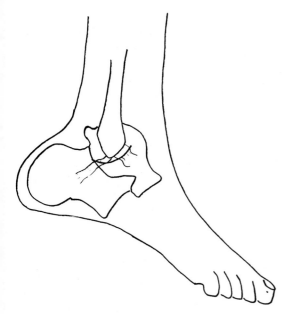

FIGURE 1.9. Placement of the incision of the capsular and lateral ankle ligaments.

avoids the lateral branches of the superficial peroneal nerve, provides better access to the calcaneofibular ligament, and can be extended to perform an anatomic reconstruction with split peroneus brevis tendon, if necessary.

4. Protect the lateral branches of the superficial peroneal nerve along the anterior extent of the incision and the sural nerve inferiorly and posteriorly as the subcutaneous tissue is incised. Palpate the talus and the tip of the fibula while passively moving the ankle to avoid inadvertently opening the subtalar joint.

5. Incise the capsule and the normally attenuated anterior talofibular and calcaneofibular ligaments 5 to 7 mm from their insertion on the fibula (Fig. 1.9). Do not transect the ligaments more than midway from their fibular attachment points. For better exposure of the calcaneofibular ligament, open the sheath and mobilize the peroneal tendons.

6. Inspect the joint. If it has not already been done arthroscopically, débride any chondral lesions and remove loose bodies.

7. Preserving the proximal fibular attachments of the capsule and anterior talofibular and calcaneofibular ligaments,

roughen the surface of the bone on the distal end of the fibula between the articular margin and the insertion of the capsule and ligaments.

8. Place two 2–0 nonabsorbable sutures in each distal ligament using a horizontal mattress weaving configuration and advance the distal ligaments to the tip of the fibula under its respective elevated proximal half. Tie the sutures on the anterior aspect while the ankle and foot are maintained in neutral flexion and slight eversion (Fig. 1.10). Next, imbricate the proximal end of each ligament over its distal end in a vest-over-pants manner.

9. Repair the peroneal tendon sheath (if opened) and the joint capsule with a 2–0 absorbable suture. If additional support for the repair is desired, mobilize the inferior extensor retinaculum from the

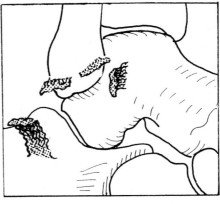

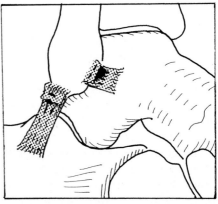

FIGURE 1.10. Suturing of the distal ligament under the proximal flap. (A) Division of anterior talofibular and calcaneofibular ligaments. (B) Suturing of the distal ligament under the proximal stumps.

sinus tarsi and imbricate it to the fibular periosteum proximal to the ligament repair (Gould et al., 1980). This maneuver requires placing the foot in maximum eversion.

10. Close the skin with interrupted 4–0 nylon suture and apply a short-leg well padded U-shaped splint to maintain the ankle and foot position.

Postoperative Management. Protected weight-bearing is used until 10 days postoperatively, at which time the splint and sutures are removed. Apply a short-leg walking cast, which is used for 6 weeks. At this point formal therapy is inititated, beginning with active ankle and subtalar motion. Resistive exercises for the peroneals and dorsiflexors, together with a tilt board for proprioceptive conditioning, are performed for the next 4 to 6 weeks. Once motion is fully restored and strength is 90 percent of the normal ankle, functional exercises including running and pivoting are allowed. The patient returns to activity usually by 3 to 4 months. Taping or an ankle orthosis is recommended for 1 year after surgery.

Anatomic Reconstruction

Anatomic reconstruction of the lateral ankle ligaments avoids limitation of subtalar motion by altering the attachment sites of the tendon graft used to reconstruct the anterior talofibular and calcaneofibular ligaments (Colville and Grondel, 1995).

Technique

1. The patient is positioned supine with a bump underneath the ipsilateral hip. With the ankle in plantarflexion, a 15 cm longitudinal incision is made centered over the posterior prominence of the lateral malleolus, extending proximally from the base of the fifth metatarsal.
2. Avoid the sural nerve, which is posterior in the incision. Open the peroneal tendon sheath and identify the peroneus brevis tendon, which lies anterior to the peroneus longus at the ankle. Remember that traction on the peroneus longus plantar-flexes the hallux metatarsal. Dissect the muscle of the peroneus brevis from the anterior two-thirds of the peroneus brevis tendon, splitting the tendon distally but leaving it attached to the base of the fifth metatarsal (Fig. 1.11A). Place a no. 2 nonabsorbable suture through the free end of the peroneus graft, using a whipstitch to taper the end of the tendon, thereby facilitating passage through the bony tunnels that are to be created.

3. A 4.5 mm drill bit is used to create the bony tunnels in the calcaneus, fibula, and talus (Fig. 1.11A). To start the transverse calcaneal tunnel, identify the origin of the calcaneofibular ligament, which lies posterior to the peroneal tendon sheath. Start the drill at a 45 degree angle to the calcaneal surface at the insertion of the calcaneofibular ligament. Distal to this point, maintaining at least a 1 cm bony bridge, start another drill hole also at a 45 degree angle, converging toward the first hole. Connect and enlarge the drill holes with a curet. From a posterior point on the fibula, posterior (deep) to the peroneal tendons and at the tip corresponding to the origin of the calcaneofibular ligament, drill a tunnel from posterior to anterior that exits at the origin of the anterior talofibular ligament. Next, drill a vertical tunnel on the neck of the talus at the insertion of the anterior talofibular ligament.

4. Before passing the tendon graft, imbricate the anterior talofibular and calcaneofibular ligaments as described in the section on delayed primary repair. Pass the tendon graft sequentially through the calcaneal, fibular, and talar tunnels (Fig. 1.11B). A commercially available curved suture passer is helpful.

5. Position the ankle in neutral and the foot in near maximum eversion. Tighten the peroneal tendon graft. Suture the graft to the calcaneofibular ligament origin and insertion first with 0 absorbable suture. Tighten the graft again, and suture the free end of the graft to the anterior talofibular limb (Fig. 1.11C).

6. Check that ankle and subtalar motion are preserved. Repair the peroneal tendon sheath at the level of the lateral malleolus with a running 2–0 absorbable suture. The tourniquet is released, and hemostasis is

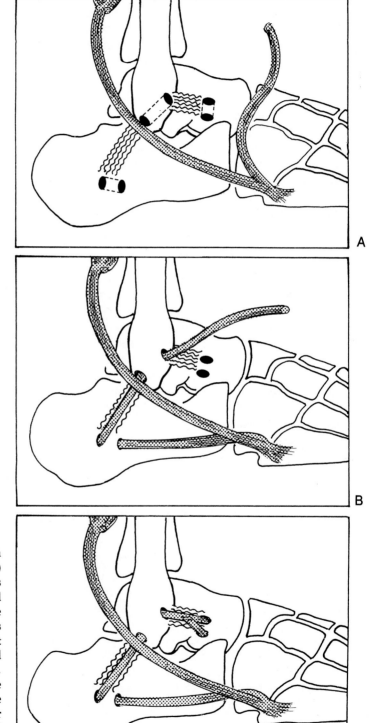

FIGURE 1.11. Anatomic reconstruction for chronic lateral ankle laxity. (A) Anterior half of the peroneus brevis tendon is harvested, leaving its distal insertion intact. Drill holes are made in the calcaneus, fibula, and talus as described in the text. (B) The split tendon is passed through the drill holes in the calcaneus and fibula, following the anatomic course of the calcaneofibular ligament. (C) The tendon is passed through the talar drill holes, following the course of the anterior talofibular ligament, and is sutured to itself.

obtained. The subcutaneous tissue is reapproximated with interrupted mattress stitches, using 2–0 absorbable suture. Close the skin with interrupted 3–0 nylon mattress stitches. A well padded, posterior splint is applied.

Postoperative Management. At 1 week remove the sutures and immobilize the ankle and foot in a short-leg cast, allowing weight-bearing as tolerated. At 6 weeks immobilization is discontinued and rehabilitation commenced according to the schedule for delayed primary repair. Most patients return to sports at 6 months. An ankle brace or orthosis is used for the first year of activity.

Syndesmosis Sprains (Distal Tibiofibular Ligament Injuries)

Syndesmosis sprains are often mistaken for lateral ankle ligament sprains until delayed recovery leads to reassessment. The major significance of these injuries includes prolonged recovery from injury, syndesmosis ossification, and diastasis of the distal tibiofibular articulation (ankle mortise). Untreated diastasis leads to symptoms of instability, loss of power with push-off, and potential degeneration of the articular surfaces of the ankle joint.

Biomechanics and Injury

The tibiofibular syndesmosis, comprised of the anterior and posterior tibiofibular ligaments, inferior transverse ligament, and interosseous ligament, stabilizes the ankle mortise. Both anterior and posterior tibiofibular ligaments demonstrate an increase in strain with ankle dorsiflexion; in addition, the anterior tibiofibular ligament undergoes lengthening during external rotation of the talus (Colville et al., 1990, 1992). Rupture of the tibiofibular syndesmosis causes diastasis, either frank or latent, of the ankle mortise (Edwards and DeLee, 1984).

Clinical Presentation

Supramalleolar tenderness and swelling are characteristic but may be obscured by later swelling that envelops the entire ankle. Tenderness of the anterior and distal tibiofibular ligaments, pain elicited by compression of the malleoli, and pain with squeezing of the mid calf are highly suggestive of injury in the absence of fracture (Hopkinson et al., 1990). Careful palpation of the lateral collateral ligaments reveals minimal or no tenderness. Talar tilt and anterior drawer test are negative.

Radiography

Anteroposterior, lateral, and mortise radiographic views are sufficient, but proximal tenderness in the calf warrants inclusion of the entire tibia and fibula in the study. Potential or latent diastasis may be missed; stress radiography is helpful for establishing the diagnosis. On the AP view the fibula should overlap the tibia by 42% of the width of the fibula and on the mortise view the separation of the fibula and tibia must not exceed 5 mm (Harper and Keller, 1989). External rotation is applied to the ankle, and an AP or mortise radiograph is obtained (Fig. 1.12).

Nonoperative Treatment

In cases without diastasis, immobilization and protection from weight-bearing are standard. Immobilization can be in the form of a bivalved cast or CAM walker, which are removed for daily therapy. Bicycling and light resistive exercises are started similar to treatment for a lateral ankle sprain. Immobilization and protection from weight-bearing are continued until unprotected walking is nonpainful and without limp.

Operative Treatment

Diastasis, frank or latent, requires treatment. Untreated diastasis causes arthrosis of the ankle, which, at the least, impairs activity. Although casting can be utilized, placement of a single, nonlagged, positional syndesmosis screw is the most reliable method.

Screw Fixation

A 3.5 mm cortical screw is used that engages both fibular cortices and only the lateral

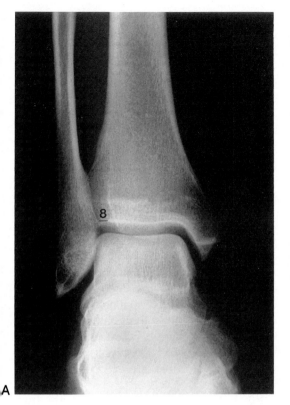 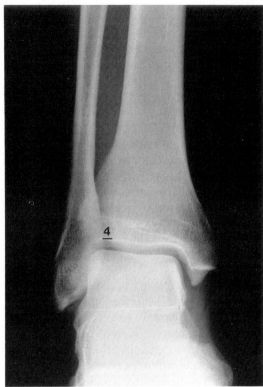

A B

FIGURE 1.12. (A) Diastasis of inferior tibiofibular articulation. (B) Normal.

cortex of the tibia 2 to 3 cm above the tibiotalar joint. Joint range of motion, soft tissue mobilization, and peroneal and dorsiflexor strengthening exercises can commence immediately after the incision is healed, at 1 week. Protected weight-bearing is used for 3 to 4 weeks. Although the screw is unlikely to break with ambulation (Kaye, 1989), it should be removed before return to sport.

Syndesmosis Ossification

Delayed return to activity because of persistent pain and weakness with push-off is frequent. It may be secondary to ossification of the tibiofibular ligaments (Fig. 1.13). If syndesmosis ossification occurs, the athlete may complain of increased "stiffness" of the leg when running and jumping. Individuals with syndesmosis ossification are at greater risk for experiencing inversion ankle sprains (Taylor et al., 1992), although excision of ossification is rarely needed.

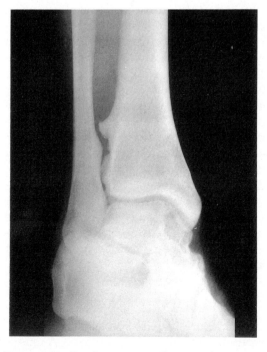

FIGURE 1.13. Syndesmosis ossification after sprain.

Ankle Fractures

Fractures of the ankle occur during both contact and noncontact sports. Primary considerations include the severity of the soft tissue component of the injury, the anatomy of the fracture, and the degree of displacement. Vigorous attention to surgical treatment and rehabilitation is necessary to avoid sport-limiting postfracture complications. Of particular importance is the need to prevent loss of ankle and subtalar motion, disturbance of ankle proprioception, and muscle weakness.

Clinical Presentation

Injury is usually dramatic. Immediate severe pain, inability to bear weight, and swelling are prominent, unless the fracture is stable, in which case limited weight-bearing may be possible. Gross deformity due to lateral talar shift can occur with fracture of both medial and lateral malleoli with associated rupture of the distal tibiofibular syndesmosis. Assessment of vascularity, sensation, and motor function of the foot is vital. Gross deformity can induce skin breakdown, especially medially, and contribute to diminished perfusion and sensation of the foot. It should be corrected by gentle longitudinal traction, even if radiography is not immediately available. Tenderness and crepitus are useful for identifying fracture location before radiographs are obtained. The entire fibula should be palpated to avoid missing a proximal fibula fracture associated with extensive syndesmosis injury. Range of motion testing is not useful for the assessment and is usually unduly painful. With delayed presentation, severe swelling and ecchymosis are usually present. Splinting and elevation should be performed as soon as possible, even if radiographs cannot be performed until transport to a hospital.

Open Fractures

Open fractures require special consideration. Wounds should not be probed. A sterile dressing soaked in iodine-povidone solution, if available, is applied to the wound; another layer of dry, sterile dressing is added, and the ankle is then placed into a well padded splint that maintains alignment. In the emergency room the wound is not reinspected. Tetanus prophylaxis and cefazolin are administered, with an aminoglycoside added for type III fractures. Cultures are not performed preoperatively.

Radiography

Anteroposterior, mortise, and lateral radiographs are usually sufficient to diagnose and classify ankle fractures. Although fractures of the medial and lateral malleolus are usually obvious, fracture of the posterior lip of the tibia (the "posterior" malleolus) and bony avulsion of the anteroinferior tibiofibular ligament may be subtle. Displacements of the malleoli, along with external rotation and shortening of the lateral malleolus, are measured.

When the medial malleolus is not fractured, deltoid ligament rupture must be considered. An increase in the articular space between the medial malleolus and medial talus, compared to the joint width between the superior talar dome and tibial plafond, confirms deltoid ligament and syndesmotic ligament rupture (Fig. 1.14). The relation of the distal tibia and fibula at the mortise normally demonstrates an overlap of the fibula and tibia on the AP view of 42% of the total width of the fibula and on the mortise view a separation, or "clear space" not exceeding 5 mm is evident (Harper and Keller, 1989). Whereas fracture of the fibula at or above the tibial plafond indicates syndesmosis injury, diagnosis of tibiofibular instability requires a demonstrable increase in distal tibiofibular separation, as seen on radiographs or by intraoperative testing.

Classification

The two major classifications are those of Lauge-Hansen (1950) and Danis-Weber (Muller et al., 1979). Lauge-Hansen classified

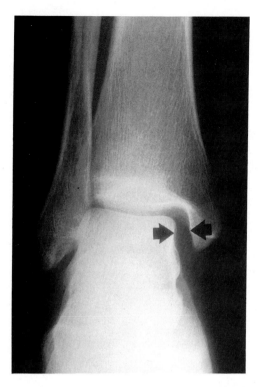

FIGURE 1.14. Lateral talar shift in mortise view (arrow), indicating deltoid ligament rupture associated with syndesmosis diastasis.

fractures based on the position of the foot and ankle and the direction of applied force. Using cadavers, he was able to demonstrate the sequence of injury that occurred. The Danis-Weber classification is based on the level of the fibular fracture as it relates to the distal tibiofibular syndesmosis (Fig. 1.15). Popularized by the AO-Group, the Danis-Weber system allows identification of those fractures (some type Bs and all type Cs) with potential tibiofibular instability. Both classification schemes are useful when formulating treatment, but the Lauge-Hansen classification, because of its detailed description, allows more accurate comparison of interstudy results.

With the Lauge-Hansen system, the foot is positioned in supination or pronation at the time of pathologic force application. Three forces are recognized: adduction, eversion, and pronation. The most frequently encountered fractures occur with the foot in supina-

tion as a result of application of either an adduction or eversion force. With the foot pronated and an abduction or eversion force applied, Lauge-Hansen noted significant syndesmotic ligament injury associated with malleolar fractures.

Indications

Nondisplaced intraarticular and minimally displaced (< 2 mm) extraarticular fractures can be treated by cast immobilization for a period of 4 to 6 weeks. Primary internal fixation is performed for all intraarticular fractures with more than 2 mm of displacement, rotation, or shortening (Joy et al., 1974). Although many supination-eversion fractures (Danis-Weber type B) can be reduced closed, the use of a long leg cast to maintain reduction, in general, is not well tolerated.

Operative Treatment

The best opportunity for restoring function of the ankle and lower extremity is anatomic reduction of the fractures accompanied by stable fixation which allows early joint motion and isometric and light resistive exercises. To this end, careful selection of incisions and minimal surgical soft tissue dissection are helpful. When possible, surgery within 12 hours is preferred before fracture swelling and blisters develop. Open fractures are operated on within 6 hours.

Technical Considerations

Fixation of the lateral malleolus is the key to restoring the mortise and correlates with outcome (Muller et al., 1979; Weber, 1993; Yablon et al., 1977). In addition, anatomic fixation of the lateral malleolus usually repositions the posterior lip fracture of the tibia by "ligamentotaxis" through the posterior tibiofibular ligament. Decisions regarding fixation of the lateral malleolus include whether to use lag screws alone or in combination with a neutralization plate, whether the plate should be lateral or posterior, and how many cortices above and below the fracture are needed for stable fixation.

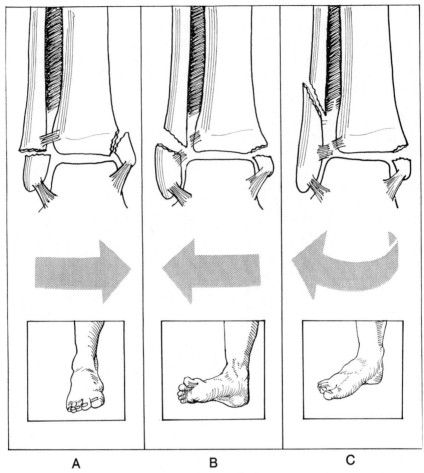

FIGURE 1.15. Danis-Weber (AO) classification of ankle fractures. (A) Type A. (B) Type B. (C) Type C.

It may be difficult to predict the method of fixation of the medial malleolus. Preferably, parallel 4.0 mm cancellous screws are used, but a tension band for comminuted fractures or a single screw may suffice. In the case of deltoid ligament rupture, the issue of whether to open the medial ankle joint remains unsettled. Although the ligament can heal without surgery (Zeegers and vander-Werken, 1989), the ankle is well visualized from the medial side, allowing irrigation and removal of traumatically produced chondral flakes from the talus, tibia, or fibula. A posterior lip fracture with more than 25% involvement of the posterior articular surface should be fixed. When the fracture has been reduced by "ligamentotaxis," an anterior to posterior lag screw is sufficient. If not, a

posteromedial incision is required to allow access to the fracture for reduction.

Currently, the most unsettled issue is when to transfix the distal tibiofibular syndesmosis (Boden, 1989). Rather than relying solely on the fracture pattern, the stability of the distal tibifibular syndesmosis is assessed by manually attempting to displace the reduced and stabilized fibula (Weber, 1993).

Fixation of Ankle Fractures

Technique

1. Under tourniquet control and with a bump placed underneath the ipsilateral hip to facilitate lateral ankle exposure, the fibula is exposed through a straight, longitudinal incision centered over the fracture. Dis-

section is carried down through the subcutaneous tissue and periosteum of the fibula without creating flaps. (This method
avoids potential injury to the sural and superficial peroneal nerves, posteriorly and
anteriorly, respectively. Gently elevate the
periosteum from the fracture ends.

2. Reduce the fibula by applying longitudinal
traction to the distal fragment with a bone
forceps or a bone hook seated in the lateral
cortex near the inferior tip. For transverse
fractures (supination-adduction or Danis-
Weber type A and pronation-eversion or
Danis-Weber type C-2 injuries), a lag
screw cannot be placed across the fracture.
In these cases, usually a one-third tubular
plate is used alone and placed laterally.
Occasionally with a Danis-Weber type A
fracture, a single axial 4.0 mm lag screw
can be inserted from the tip into the canal
of the fibula. With the most common ankle
fractures, Weber-Danis types B and C-1,
the fibular fracture is oblique in the AP
plane. If the fracture length is at least two
times the diameter of the fibula, lag screws
alone (usually two or three) are inserted
perpendicular to the fracture. Otherwise, a
single AP lag screw and a laterally placed
one-third tubular plate are used (Fig. 1.16).
A posterior gliding plate which can be helpful in osteopenic bone, may cause irritation
of the peroneal tendons and should be
avoided (Schaffer and Manoli, 1987). If a lag
screw has been used, a minimum of four
cortices distally and four cortices proximally should be sufficient to stabilize the
fracture. If lag screw fixation is not possible,
fixation should include six cortices proximally and four cortices distally.

3. If further reduction of a posterior lip fracture of the tibia is not necessary, as confirmed by postfixation radiographs after
fibular stabilization, the medial malleolus
is exposed by a straight, longitudinal incision centered over its tip. Dissection is
performed straight down to the malleolus
and the periosteum elevated from the
edges. To visualize the joint, open the
capsule at the junction of the medial malleolus and the plafond. Protect and do not

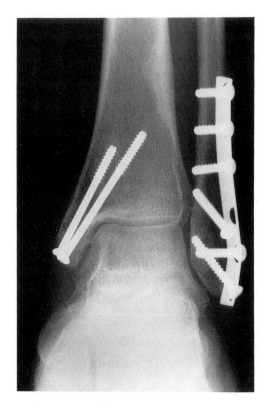

FIGURE 1.16. Internal fixation of Danis-Weber type
B ankle fracture.

ligate the saphenous vein. Inspect and
irrigate the joint.

4. Use bone forceps or a tenaculum to obtain
and maintain reduction of the medial malleolus, as provisional K-wires may interfere with placement of permanent fixation.
Use the AO small fragment parallel drill
guide to insert two 4.0 mm cancellous
screws. An intraoperative mortise radiograph should demonstrate that the screws
do not pass into the joint.

5. If after fibular fixation a posterior lip fracture is not reduced, the medial incision
must be altered to expose the fracture. In
this circumstance, make an incision along
the posteromedial border of the tibia and
medial malleolus, following the curve of
the posterior tibial tendon. A bone forceps
or tenaculum can be used to reduce the
posterior lip fracture and maintain it while
fixation from the anterior position is
performed.

6. Fixation of the posterior lip fracture is by a 4.0 mm lag screw inserted from anterior to posterior through a short vertical incision immediately above the distal tibial articular surface (plafond) and along the medial border of the anterior tibial tendon. Drill and insert the lag screw with slight lateral displacement of the anterior tibial tendon. If the threads of the lag screw are too long and cross the fracture, cut the threads short with a wire cutter.

7. Evaluate the stability of the tibiofibular syndesmosis after all fractures have been satisfactorily fixed. Using a bone hook, attempt to displace the fibula laterally. If no instability is present, a syndesmosis screw is unnecessary. If instability is present, however, the syndesmosis must be stabilized. Care must be taken to avoid narrowing the syndesmosis by performing syndesmosis fixation with the ankle in neutral and using a noncompressive screw. Insert a fully tapped, 3.5 mm cortical screw parallel to the ankle joint just above the distal tibiofibular ligaments (2–3 cm above the joint). Engage both fibular and only the lateral tibial cortices (Fig. 1.17).

8. Obtain final radiographs, and close the wounds in layers. Drains are usually unnecessary. Apply a well padded U-splint (medial and lateral stirrups with a plantar foot plate) that maintains the ankle and foot in neutral.

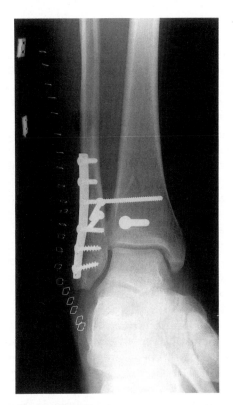

FIGURE 1.17. Syndesmosis stabilization.

Postoperative Management

Elevation is crucial to minimize swelling postoperatively. Non-weight-bearing ambulation is used routinely. At 1 week the sutures are removed. Either a short-leg cast with the dorsal portion anterior to the ankle and foot removed to allow active ankle dorsiflexion or a commercial CAM walker with the ankle set at neutral is applied and worn at all times except when therapy and ankle range of motion exercises are being performed. Ankle support is necessary to prevent loss of dorsiflexion during the early postoperative period.

Initial therapy consists in passive and active ankle range-of-motion exercises, electrical stimulation, icing and whirlpool bath to reduce swelling, and light resistive exercises with surgical tubing. No weight-bearing is allowed for 4 weeks. If a syndesmosis screw has been used, non-weight-bearing is maintained for 6 weeks. Thereafter, partial weight-bearing is started, even for fractures requiring stabilization of the syndesmosis. Full weight-bearing is allowed at 6 to 8 weeks after radiographs demonstrate early healing. If used, a syndesmosis screw is removed under local anesthesia at 8 weeks. Running on a treadmill can usually begin by 8 to 10 weeks. Lateral slides, figure-of-eight running, and ankle proprioception training on a tilt board are important before attempting unrestricted running and sport specific training. Many athletes can return to sports by 4 months.

Prolonged soft tissue swelling and hardware intolerance, because of the superficial location of the fracture, are frequent. When possible, removal of fracture implants is delayed until after the season. All hardware can be removed at 4 months, with a short recovery of 1 to 2 weeks thereafter.

Osteochondral Lesions of the Talus

An osteochondral lesion of the talar dome (Fig. 1.18) is a significant cause of persistent pain after ankle injury. This disorder of the ankle was first described in 1922 by Kappis. He theorized that the problem was due to spontaneous necrosis of the talar dome. Berndt and Harty in 1959 termed these lesions "transchondral fractures" because they could be created traumatically. Trauma is the most commonly accepted etiology for these lesions, though with the development of computed tomography (CT) and MRI scanning it has been found that some defects are due to spontaneuos necrosis of the bone (Loomer et al., 1993).

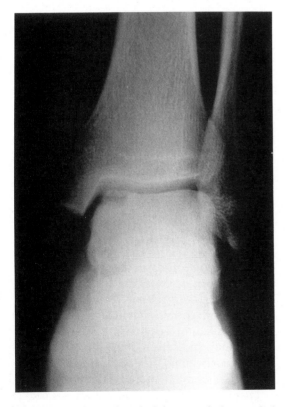

FIGURE 1.18. Osteochondral lesion of the medial talar dome.

Pathogenesis

Berndt and Harty (1959) advanced the understanding of this condition through a clinical series and cadaveric studies that demonstrated the pathomechanics of the injury. Their bench studies corroborated the clinical impression that these lesions follow two distinct patterns. Those located on the lateral talar dome are usually anterior, and those on the medial side are found at the apex or on the posterior dome. Both types of lesions have been produced in cadavers by application of a loading force through the leg onto an ankle fixed in inversion. When the inverted ankle was dorsiflexed, the result was an anterolateral lesion. A posteromedial lesion was created when the inverted ankle was in plantarflexion and similarly loaded.

In dorsiflexion the wider anterior half of the talar dome fits tightly in the mortise. With an excessive inverting force, the talus rotates laterally in the frontal plane causing the lateral margin of the talus to impact and compress the articular surface of the fibula. This maneuver produces a small area of indentation in the talar margin. If the talar rotation continues, the margin of the talar dome can be sheared off.

Conversely, when the ankle is in plantarflexion the narrow posterior half of the talus fits loosely in the mortise. Inversion of the talus causes the talus to rock laterally and the medial border impacts the articular surface of the tibia. External rotation of the tibia produces grinding against the medial talar ridge, an action whose force is increased as the collateral ligaments of the ankle tighten. It leads to a defect in the posteromedial dome.

Classification

Berndt and Harty (1959) developed a classification scheme based on the degree of displacement of the defect (Fig. 1.19). Stage I describes compression of the cartilage and underlying bone. A stage II lesion has a partially detached fragment of bone and cartilage. A stage III lesion is completely detached, but it remains in its bone bed,

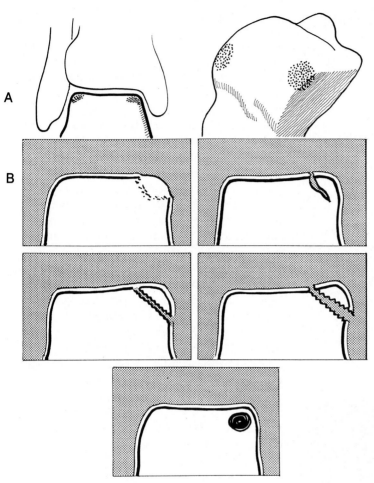

FIGURE 1.19. Location and classification of osteochondral lesions of the talus. (A) Lateral lesions tend to be anterior, whereas medial lesions are more posterior. (B) Classification: stages I, II, III, IV, and V (or IIa).

whereas a stage IV lesion has become displaced.

This classification scheme is still commonly used but has been modified to include a newly described lesion (Anderson et al., 1989; Loomer, et al., 1993). The use of CT and MRI scanning has allowed identification of a subchondral lesion in the talar dome as a fifth type of talar dome lesion. Although this lesion may occur by spontaneous necrosis, it has been observed to occur after documented stage I and II lesions. It is thought to be due to resorption of necrotic bone, which then leaves a rim of sclerotic bone filled with fluid. It has been termed a stage IIa or stage V lesion (Loomer, et al., 1993; Thompson and Loomer, 1984).

Further characterization of the medial and lateral lesions show that in general those on the medial side tend to be deep with a cup-shaped base, whereas lateral lesions are

often shallow or wafer-shaped. Moreover, 98% of the lateral lesions have a definite history of associated trauma, whereas that is true for only 70% of the medial lesions (Canale and Belding, 1980; Flick and Gould, 1985).

Clinical Presentation

The athlete presents with a complaint of ankle pain that can be localized to the medial or lateral side. The pain may be constant or associated with certain activities. Some patients notice "catching" or locking of the ankle, which may indicate a stage III or IV loose fragment. Swelling may occur but is not common. Loss of ankle motion is also unusual.

There is usually a history of an ankle sprain, although it may have occurred in the distant past. An unfortunate feature of these injuries is that they are often not recognized

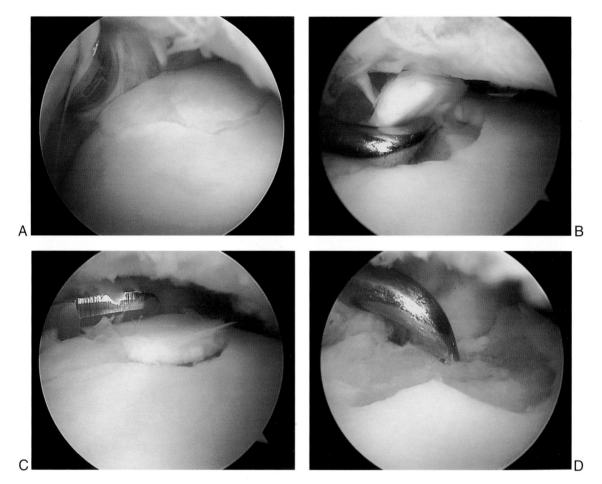

FIGURE 1A–D. OCD of anterolateral talar dome (A). The cartilage flap retains only a small hinge and is devoid of attached subchondral bone (B). Resection of flap (C) and microfracture of bony bed of talus using special awl (D) to stimulate fibrocartilage ingrowth.

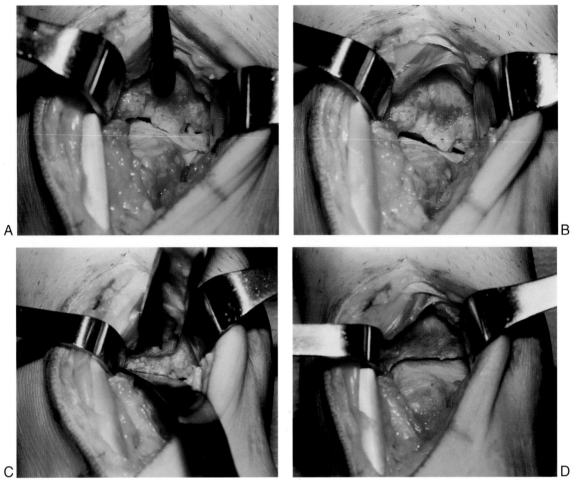

FIGURE 2A–D. Open debridement of ankylosed ankle after open talar dislocation. Exposure is medial to anterior tibial tendon through initial open wound. Anterior capsule has been elevated and retracted to show anterior tibial spur (A). Attempted dorsiflexion causes impingement of spur on talus (B). Osteotomy of spur with malleable retractor protecting talar dome (C). Post-debridement appearance (D).

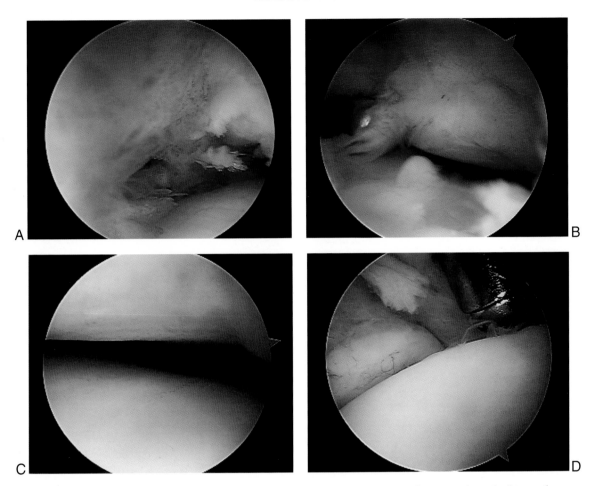

FIGURE 3A–D. Post-traumatic synovitis (A,B). After debridement note the smooth articular surfaces (C,D).

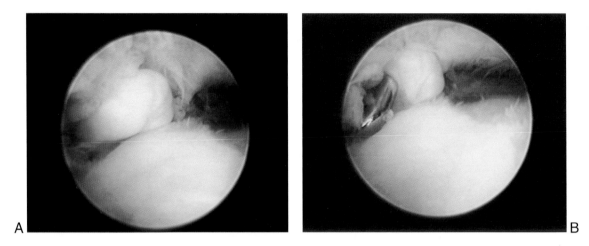

FIGURE 4A,B. Loose body in degenerative ankle adjacent to medial malleolus. Note the chondral wear along the dome of the talus, immediately beneath the tibial plafond.

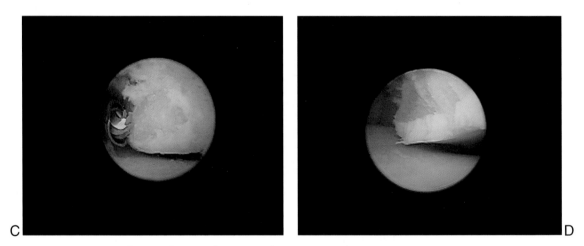

FIGURE 4C,D. Arthroscopic debridement of anterior tibial spur.

when they occur (Flick and Gould, 1985; Burkas et al., 1982; Loomer et al., 1993).

Radiography

In most cases a careful review of the routine radiographs of the ankle demonstrates the lesion. Misinterpretation of radiographs has been shown to be a real problem when evaluating these lesions, as some of the lesions are not visible on standard radiographs. Careful review of serial radiographs may show that in some cases the lesion becomes radiographically apparent only after some months (Flick and Gould, 1985).

If clinical suspicion is not verified by the plain films, a technetium bone scan is a sensitive test to undertake as the next step. The bone scan shows an area of increased tracer uptake in the region of the talus corresponding to the lesion. It is not useful for characterizing the lesion further, however, or for describing the stage of the lesion.

Computed tomography can provide a more detailed picture of the lesion and can accurately determine the size of the lesion (Anderson et al., 1989; Loomer et al., 1993). It gives no information, though, about the de-gree of overlying cartilage damage. It may not identify a stage I lesion, but it can show the progression of a stage I or II lesion to a subchondral cyst. If the lesion has been satisfactorily identified on plain radiographs, it is not necessary to obtain a CT scan.

Magnetic resonance imaging detects changes that occur in the bone marrow due to a fracture and is a sensitive test for all stages of osteochondral lesions (Fig. 1.20) (Anderson et al., 1989). The marrow normally has a high signal intensity on both T1- and T2-weighted images due to the presence of fat. After a fracture there is a decrease in the T1 signal intensity due at first to the presence of edema and later to the formation of fibrous tissue. The extent of edema may be much greater than the extent of the lesion, a situation that can lead to overestimating the size of the lesion. There are also reports of MRI discovering abnormalities that are asymptomatic, so the study must be interpreted with the clinical circumstances in mind.

Nonoperative Treatment

The initial nonoperative treatment consists in rest, oral antiinflammatory medications,

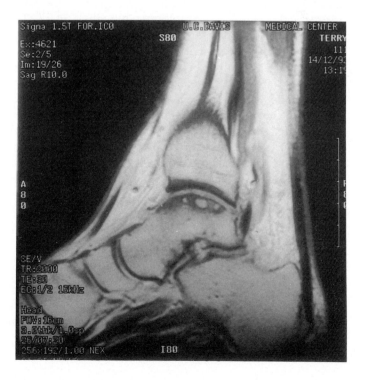

FIGURE 1.20. MRI of an osteochondral lesion of the talar dome.

casting, and non-weight-bearing. Canale and Belding (1980) recommended initial nonoperative treatment for all stage I and II lesions and for medial stage III lesions. They believed that lateral stage III and all stage IV lesions required early excision. Operative treatment is indicated for athletes with lower grade lesions who fail nonoperative treatment. The length of time that nonoperative measures should be pursued varies depending on the duration of symptoms and the athlete's demands and expectations.

Operative Treatment

For higher grade lesions and lesions that do not respond to nonoperative measures, surgical intervention is necessary (Anderson et al., 1989; Canale and Belding, 1980; Davidson et al., 1967; Mukherjee and Young, 1973; Naumetz and Schweigel, 1980; Yvars, 1976). The essential treatment is to excise the lesion and drill its base to promote revascularization and formation of a repair cartilage. There are variations on how it may be accomplished depending on the location, accessibility of the lesion, and its stage. Lateral lesions were traditionally approached through an anterior arthrotomy, but the development of ankle arthroscopy has offered a minimally invasive technique particularly suited to treating these anterior lesions (Ferkel and Scranton, 1993; Martin et al., 1989; Parisien, 1986; Parisien and Vangsness, 1985; Pritsch et al., 1986; Van Buecken et al., 1989). After removing any loose fragments the base of the defect can be drilled under arthroscopic visualization with a small drill point or K-wire.

Arthroscopy is also used for medial lesions, but the more posterior location of these defects makes access with instruments difficult (Ferkel and Scranton, 1993; Martin et al., 1989; Parisien, 1986; Parisien and Vangsness, 1985; Pritsch et al., 1986; Van Buecken et al., 1989). Ferkel and Scranton (1993) described the use of a transmalleolar portal for drilling medial lesions after excision and curettage has been performed

through standard anterolateral and anteromedial ports. Instruments have been devised that can aid in triangulating the defect through the malleolus. Free-hand drilling with a small K-wire through the medial malleolus can also be done.

Open techniques can be used for large lateral lesions and are useful for many medial ones. Stage IV lesions that are large may be replaced and fixed with a K-wire, Herbert screw, or absorbable pin (Pettine and Morrey, 1987). Stage IIA or V subchondral cysts or other lesions with an intact overlying cartilage can be approached from the adjacent gutter, elevating the cartilage and allowing the defect to be curetted and drilled (Lian and Marder, 1994). Bone graft may be placed into the defect, with the cartilage placed back over the defect and held in place with an absorbable pin. The lateral lesions can be approached with an anterolateral arthrotomy. The medial lesions are usually approached through a transmalleolar osteotomy that has been predrilled and pretapped. Other approaches to medial lesions include the anterior approach to the malleolus under the anterior tibialis tendon and the posterior approach to the malleolus through the posterior tibialis tendon sheath (Flick and Gould, 1985; Loomer et al., 1993).

Although the results of treatment, arthroscopic or open, are generally favorable (Alexander and Lichtman, 1980), some studies have indicated that patients may develop significant ankle problems. Canale and Belding (1980) found that 50% of their patients, whether treated surgically or conservatively, had radiographic evidence of ankle arthrosis at an average follow-up of 11.2 years. Pettine and Morrey (1987) found radiographic evidence of arthritis at a 7 year follow-up in 41% of patients with type I or II lesions and in 46% of those with type III or IV lesions. Scharling (1978) found that only half of his patients were pain-free, and that limited ankle motion was present in 37% of patients 7 years after treatment. He also reported that there was radiographic evidence of degenerative changes in 40% of the patients.

Arthroscopic Drilling of Lateral Talar Dome Lesion

Technique

1. A general anesthetic is provided and a tourniquet applied. The ankle is infiltrated with 10 cc of 0.5% bupivacaine (Marcaine) with epinephrine.
2. Standard anteromedial and anterolateral portals are made and the joint inspected. The lesion is identified, with disrupted or soft cartilage overlying the defect on the lateral talar dome.
3. The disrupted cartilage surface is débrided with a small curet and a shaver. Any loose osteocartilaginous fragments are removed.
4. The base of the defect is drilled with an 0.062 inch K-wire passed through the lateral portal while visualizing it through the arthroscope in the medial portal (Fig. 1.21). Additional passes of the K-wire can be made directly through the skin into the defect so the defect is drilled in multiple directions.
5. The tourniquet is released, and bleeding vessels are identified diffusely in the base of the defect.

Postoperative Management

The athlete is kept non-weight-bearing on crutches for 4 to 6 weeks. The skin sutures are removed at 7 to 10 days. Ankle motion exercises are started immediately, but continuous passive motion devices are not used. Formal therapy for assisted range-of-motion exercises, modalities to decrease swelling and pain (interferential stimulation, intermittent compression, whirlpool), and isometric exercises are often helpful. At 6 to 8 weeks, once pain-free weight-bearing is accomplished, proprioceptive training with a tilt board and full resistive exercises are started. The ability to perform functional exercises is necessary before return to sports, which averages 3 months.

Open Treatment of Medial Talar Dome Lesions

Surgical Technique

1. A general anesthetic is provided and a thigh tourniquet applied. The iliac crest is prepared for a bone graft. A 5 cm longitudinal incision is made over the medial malleolus, and the tip of the malleolus is exposed subperiosteally.
2. The malleolus is predrilled and tapped for two 4.0 mm cancellous screws.
3. A medial malleolar osteotomy is made with the oscillating saw at the level of the tibial plafond. A slight chevron shape to the osteotomy ensures that it can be re-

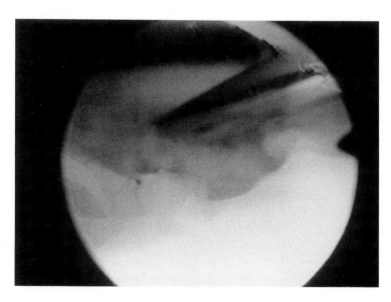

FIGURE 1.21. Arthroscopic drilling of a medial dome lesion fixation with K-wire.

placed anatomically. The malleolus is reflected distally on the fibers of the deltoid ligament, exposing the medial side of the talus.

4. If the lesion is small or the overlying cartilage disrupted, the cartilage is débrided and the defect in the bone curetted and then drilled with multiple passes with a 0.062 inch K-wire.

5. If the lesion is large and can be replaced, the base is curetted (Fig. 1.22) and drilled with a 0.062 inch K-wire. The osteocartilaginous lesion is then replaced in its bed and fixed with one or two absorbable polyglycolic acid pins or Herbert screws.

6. If the lesion is large and cannot be replaced but the overlying cartilage is intact, the cartilage is elevated with a Freer elevator. The lesion is approached from the side of the talus in the gutter. The underlying defect in the bone is curetted and drilled with a 0.062 inch K-wire. A cancellous bone graft is obtained from the exposed tibia at the malleolar osteotomy site or from the iliac crest. The graft is inserted into the defect and the cartilage replaced over it and fixed with one or two absorbable polyglycolic acid pins or small screws.

7. The malleolus is then replaced and fixed with two 4.0 mm cancellous screws. The skin is closed and a posterior splint applied.

8. Weight-bearing is not allowed for 6 weeks. The skin sutures are removed after 10 to 14 days, and a removable orthosis is worn to protect the osteotomy. As soon as the wound allows, active ankle motion exercises are performed. Formal therapy is not started until the osteotomy has healed (usually 4–6 weeks). Thereafter therapy progresses as described above with patients requiring a minimum of 4 months to return to impact sports.

Posterior Ankle Pain

Pain from the posterior aspect of the ankle has been called posterior impingement or talar compression syndrome (Brodsky and Khalil, 1986; Hamilton, 1982, 1993; Quirk, 1982; Wredmark et al., 1991). The variety of injuries that cause pain in this area include fracture of the medial talar tubercle, symptomatic os trigonum, tenosynovitis of the flexor hallucis longus, posterior ankle or subtalar joint impingement, and subtalar tarsal coalition.

Posterior ankle pain must be distinguished from disorders of the Achilles tendon. The posterior ankle joint, ligaments, and flexor tendons passing through this area are located much deeper than the Achilles tendon, which is superficial and easily palpable. In

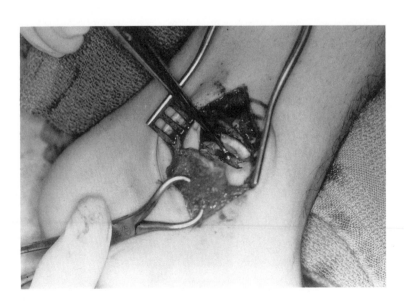

FIGURE 1.22. Open treatment of an osteochondral lesion of the medial talar dome. The medial malleolus has been osteotomized and reflected distally. The cartilage over the defect has been elevated, and a curet is used to débride the lesion prior to bone grafting.

addition, most Achilles tendon conditions are caused by dorsiflexion injuries, whereas posterior ankle injuries are usually caused by plantarflexion. Therefore a careful history and physical examination allow the physician to discriminate between these anatomic sites.

Anatomy

The posterior half of the talar dome slopes inferiorly, and the underlying surface of the posterior facet of the subtalar joint rises posteriorly. There is a small nonarticular area between these two joints from which two bony tubercles extend. The posteromedial tubercle is continuous with the medial talar surface. Fibers of the deltoid ligament attach to it. It is occasionally involved as part of a medial subtalar coalition (Hamilton, 1993; Paulos et al., 1983).

The posterolateral tubercle is larger and may be prominent. Its undersurface has articular cartilage and is in continuity with the posterior facet of the subtalar joint. It provides an origin for most of the ligamentous attachments on the posterior talus. The posterior talofibular ligament, a strong, horizontally directed band that connects to the lateral malleolus, attaches to its superior surface. The fibulotalocalcaneal ligament attaches to its medial surface, and the posterior talocalcaneal ligament attaches inferiorly (Hamilton, 1993; Paulos et al., 1983).

In 3% to 13% of the population there is an accessory bone associated with the posterolateral tubercle, the os trigonum (Brodsky and Khalil, 1986; Paulos et al., 1983; Quirk, 1982). It develops from an accessory center of ossification and appears between the ages of 8 to 10 years (Brodsky and Khalil, 1986). It may articulate with the posterolateral process by either a synovial joint or a fibrous synchondrosis. The ligamentous attachments to the posterolateral tubercle also extend onto the os trigonum.

The two posterior tubercles define the sulcus for the tendon of the flexor hallucis longus muscle. The fibroosseous canal of the flexor tendon is directed inferiorly, medially, and anteriorly. Its floor is covered with fibers of the posterior talofibular ligament, and

overlying the tendon sheath is the flexor retinaculum.

Posterior Ankle Impingement

Posterior ankle impingement (Fig. 1.23) occurs during maximum plantarflexion of the ankle when the posterolateral tubercle of the talus is caught between the undersurface of the tibia above and the superior surface of the calcaneus below (Howse, 1982). Pain is caused by compression of the interposed capsule and synovium of the ankle, the subtalar joints, or both (Quirk, 1982). This condition is more likely to appear in the presence of a trigonal process or an os trigonum, both of which are bulky, bony projections, although in most cases these prominences are asymptomatic (Hamilton, 1993). This disorder has been described in those who undertake ballet and theatrical dancing, soccer, and downhill running (Brodsky, 1986; Hardaker et al., 1985; Hedrick and McBryde, 1994).

The posterior process of the talus can be fractured during forced plantarflexion injury by one of two mechanisms. The fracture may be due to compression from the posterior lip of the tibia, the posterior calcaneus, or both (Paulos et al., 1983). This mechanism is responsible for posterior ankle soft tissue impingement. The other mechanism of fracture is an avulsion injury caused by tension through its various ligamentous attachments (Hamilton, 1993).

Clinical Presentation

These injuries present as either an acute event or with gradual onset as the result of recurrent repetitive trauma. The examination demonstrates deep palpable tenderness in the interval between the Achilles tendon and the talus. Stressed plantarflexion is usually painful as well (Paulos et al.,1983; Veazey et al., 1992).

Radiography

The evaluation should include routine radiographs of the foot and ankle. In addition, a lateral radiograph of the ankle in maximum plantarflexion can indicate bony impingement posteriorly. The lateral radiograph may

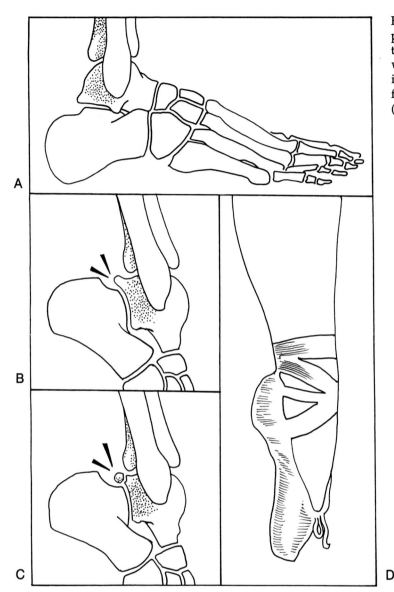

FIGURE 1.23. Posterior ankle impingement (A) The ankle in neutral. (B) Posterior impingement with plantarflexion. (C) Posterior impingement with os trigonum or fracture of the trigonal process. (D) Ballerina's foot en pointe.

ment posteriorly. The lateral radiograph may indicate an os trigonum or fracture of the trigonal process. A fracture generally exhibits irregular edges, whereas an os trigonum is smooth, although this differentiation be difficult to determine on standard radiographs. In questionable cases a bone scan can be confirmatory of fracture (Fig. 1.24) (Paulos et al., 1983; Veazey et al., 1992).

Nonoperative Treatment

The initial treatment of posterior soft tissue impingement is activity limitation until symptoms resolve. This step can be achieved with a short-leg walking orthosis for 2 to 3 weeks if there is significant, acute pain. NSAIDs may relieve symptoms due to acute inflammation, and a single corticosteroid injection into the posterior ankle structures may help for resistant cases (see below).

An acute fracture of the posterior process should be immobilized in a short-leg walking cast for 4 weeks, followed by 2 to 4 weeks in a removable walking orthosis. Gentle ankle motion exercises are then started. If symptoms persist, immobilization is repeated for a longer duration, or the fragment is excised.

FIGURE 1.24. Bone scan of an os trigonum fracture.

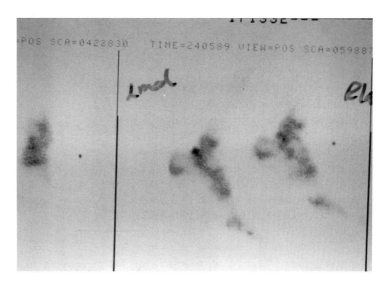

The injection technique for posterior ankle pain is as follows.

1. A diagnostic injection uses an equal mixture of 3 ml of 1.0% lidocaine and 0.5% bupivacaine without epinephrine. A therapeutic injection is the same, but after injection of the local anesthetic 0.5 to 1.0 ml of a steroid preparation is injected through the same needle.
2. The local anesthetic is injected through a 25 gauge 1.5 inch needle placed just posterior to the peroneal tendons on the lateral side of the ankle. The site of entrance is at the level of the anterior ankle joint, which can be readily located. The needle is directed obliquely toward the center of the posterior ankle. The tip is used as a probe to identify the distal tibia, talus, and calcaneus, and the local anesthetic is injected at about the level of the talus.
3. If the injection is for diagnostic purposes only, the needle is then removed, and the patient's response to provocative maneuvers of forced plantar flexion are noted over the following 5 to 10 minutes. The patient is asked to record his or her response over the ensuing 3 to 4 hours.
4. If the injection is therapeutic, the needle is left in place; and the cortisone solution in a second syringe is injected through the same needle.

Operative Treatment

Surgical treatment is reserved for those athletes who do not obtain adequate relief with nonoperative means. Fracture of the posterior process or a large symptomatic os trigonum are easily excised through a posterior medial approach. It is safest to approach the posterior ankle medially because the neurovascular bundle can be protected. Laterally, the sural nerve is susceptible to irritation, even when gentle retraction is used. In cases of unrelieved soft tissue impingement, a section of the posterior capsule of the ankle is excised and any large prominence of the posterior talar tubercle removed as well. These procedures generally allow complete return to dance and athletic activities without further problems (Brodsky and Khalil, 1986; Hamilton, 1993; Hardaker, 1989; Hedrick and McBryde, 1994; Howse, 1982; Paulos et al., 1983; Quirk, 1982; Veazey et al., 1992).

Correction of Posterior Ankle Impingement

Technique

1. A general anesthetic is provided and a thigh tourniquet applied. A bump is placed under the opposite hip to facilitate exposure of the medial side of the posterior ankle.

2. A longitudinal curved incision is made in line with the flexor tendons posterior to the medial malleolus. The flexor retinaculum is divided in line with the incision, and the flexor digitorum longus tendon is identified by dorsiflexing the toes. The dissection continues along the interval between the flexor digitorum longus tendon and the posterior tibial artery, which is posterior to the tendon.
3. With the neurovascular bundle gently retracted posteriorly and the flexor digitorum longus tendon retracted anteriorly, the underlying flexor hallucis longus (FHL) tendon is observed intimately applied to the posterior ankle. Dorsiflexion of the great toe helps to identify its tendon. The tunnel through which it passes into the foot is defined lateral to the tendon by the trigonal process.
4. Once the trigonal process or os trigonum has been identified, it is removed by sharp dissection, being careful to cut against the bone and not injure the FHL tendon. A small rongeur can smooth the remaining bone if there is a fractured process.
5. If the cause of pain is believed to be soft tissue impingement, the posterior ankle and subtalar joint caspules should be opened and a segment of posterior capsule removed from each.
6. The wound is closed in layers with repair of the flexor retinaculum using interrupted 2–0 absorbable sutures. After closing the skin, a posterior splint is applied to the leg and foot.

Postoperative Management. The patient is kept non-weight-bearing on crutches for 10 to 14 days. The skin sutures are then removed, and weight-bearing is allowed to progress as tolerated. Range of motion exercises are started as soon as possible. Formal therapy for resistive exercises and proprioceptive training are begun at 4 to 6 weeks. Activities are then allowed as tolerated.

Tibiotalar Spurs

Often the result of cumulative microtrauma, bone spurs involving the ankle can produce pain and limitation of motion with sport. When these degenerative exostoses affect only a small area of the joint (e.g., the anterior margin), excision by open or arthroscopic surgery is usually curative in the symptomatic athlete.

Mechanism of Injury

Spurs are multifactorial in origin. Avulsion of ligaments leads to ossicles, which usually are found adjacent to the lateral and medial malleoli. Anterior marginal spurs (Fig. 1.25), although occasionally caused by an acute impact leading to later spur formation, are usually the result of repetitive dorsiflexion stresses associated with sports (O'Donoghue, 1957). Athletes participating in basketball, soccer, and dancing are particularly prone to develop these changes (Kleiger, 1988; O'Donoghue, 1957).

Clinical Presentation

Many anterior tibiotalar spurs are asymptomatic or minimally symptomatic. In some patients, however, mechanical impingement occurs as the tibia rolls forward over the talus, causing pain and weakness during push-off, thereby limiting activity (O'Donoghue, 1957). Physical findings include local-

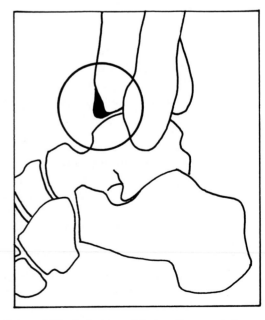

FIGURE 1.25. Anterior ankle impingement from a distal tibial spur.

FIGURE 1.26. Anterior tibiotalar spur with fragmentation.

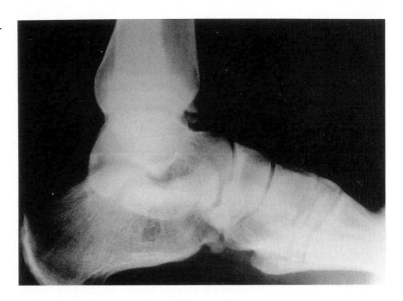

ized anterior joint tenderness, palpable
osteophyte formation, and occasionally synovial thickening and limited dorsiflexion.

Patients with medial or lateral ossicles may
complain of pain about the affected malleolus
associated with localized tenderness. Especially with lateral ossicles, examination
should document any associated lateral instability. If the ossicles are intraarticular, there
may be complaints of locking or a sensation
of a "joint mouse."

Radiography

Routine radiography is usually sufficient to
diagnose the presence of osteophytes along
the anterior tibiotalar joint and plan any
resection (Fig. 1.26). However, it may be

difficult to determine from these studies if the
medial and lateral ossicles are extraarticular
or intraarticular. Arthrography, MRI, or arthroscopy may be needed in these cases.

Treatment

Many symptomatic patients respond to nonoperative measures, such as antiinflammatory agents and shoe modification, including
heel elevation for anterior tibiotalar spurs. If
symptoms persist, the lesion is surgically
exicised. Arthroscopic or open treatment of
tibiotalar spurs involves resection primarily
of the anterior tibial lip to allow improved
talar excursion with full dorsiflexion, which is
confirmed at surgery (Fig. 1.27). Large spurs

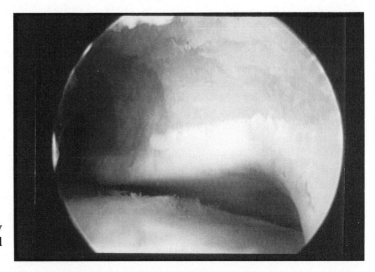

FIGURE 1.27. Arthroscopic view
after excision of an anterior tibial
spur.

on the talar neck should also be removed, but small lesions can be left alone, provided adequate clearance on the tibia has been obtained. Medial and lateral ossicles entangled in the collateral ligaments are often more easily removed by a small incision than by arthroscopic techniques.

Postoperative Management

The ankle and foot are immobilized briefly in a well-padded posterior or U-splint until the wounds are healed at 1 week. Therapeutic ankle motion, active and passive, is then undertaken in conjunction with modalities to minimize swelling and pain. Stationary cycling and swimming are encouraged to maximize recovery as soon as the wounds are healed. Strengthening programs are started once motion is regained. Most athletes return to sports by 2 months.

References

Alexander AH, Lichtman DM: Surgical treatment of transchondral talar-dome fractures (osteochondritis dissecans): long-term follow-up. Bone Joint Surg Am 62:646–652, 1980

Anderson IF, Crichton KJ, Grattan-Smith T, et al: Osteochondral fractures of the dome of the talus. Bone Joint Surg Am 71:1143–1152, 1989

Anderson KJ, Lecocq JF, Lecocq EA: Recurrent anterior subluxation of the ankle joint: a preliminary report of two cases and an experimental study. J Bone Joint Surg Am 34:853–860, 1952

Barrett JE, Tanji JL, Drake C. et al: High- versus low-top shoes for the prevention of ankle sprains in basketball players: a prospective randomized study. Am J Sports Med 21:582–585, 1993

Bassett FH III, Gates HS, Billys JB, et al: Talar impingement by the anteroinferior tibiofibular ligament. J Bone Joint Surg Am 72:55–59, 1990

Berndt AL, Harty M: Transchondral fractures (oesteochrondritis dissecans) of the talus. Bone Joint Surg Am 41:988–1020, 1959

Black HM, Brand RL, Eichelberger MF: An improved technique for the evaluation of ligamentous injury in severe ankle sprains. Am J Sports Med 6:276–282, 1978

Boden SD, Labropoulos PA, McCowin P, et al: Mechanical considerations for the syndes-

mosis screw: a cadaver study. J Bone Joint Surg Am 71:1548–1555, 1989

Boruta PM, Bishop, JO, Braly WG, et al: Acute lateral ankle ligament injuries: a literature review. Food Ankle 11:107–113, 1990

Brodsky AE, Khalil MA: Talar compression syndrome. Am J Sports Med 14:472–476, 1986

Brostrom L: Sprained ankles. I. Anatomic lesions in recent sprains. Acta Chir Scand 128:483–495, 1964

Brostom L: Sprained ankles. VI. Surgical treatment of "chronic" ligament ruptures. Acta Chir Scand 132:551–565, 1966

Burks, RT, Morgan J: Anatomy of the lateral ankle ligaments. Am J Sports Med 22:72–77, 1994

Burkus JK, Sella EJ, Scuthwick WD: Occult injuries of the talus diagnosed by bone scan and tomography. Foot ANkle 4:316–324, 1982

Canale ST, Belding, EH: Osteochrondral lesions of the talus. Bone Joint Surg Am 62:97–102, 1980

Chrisman OD, Snook GA: Reconstruction of the lateral ligament tears of the ankle: an experimental study and clinical evaluation of seven patients treated by a new modification of the Elmslie procedure. J Bone Joint Surg Am 51:904–912, 1969

Colville MR, Grondel RJ: Anatomic reconstruction of the lateral ankle ligaments using a split peroneus brevis tendon graft. Am J Sports Med 23:210–213, 1995

Colville MR, Marder RA, Boyle JJ, et al: Strain measurement in lateral ankle ligaments. Am J Sports Med 18:196–200, 1990

Colville MR, Marder RA, Zarins B: Reconstruction of the lateral ankle ligaments: a biomechanical analysis. Am J Sports Med 20:594–600, 1992

Davidson AM, Steele, HD, MacKenzie DA, Penny JA: A review of twenty-one cases of transchondral fracture of the talus. J Trauma 7:378–414, 1967

Dehne E: Die Klinik der frischen und habituellen Adduktionssupinationsdistorsion des Fusses. Dtsch Z 242:40–61, 1934

Dias LD: The lateral ankle sprain: an experimental study. J Trauma 19:266–269, 1979

Edwards GS Jr, DeLee JC: Ankle diastasis without fracture. Food Ankle 4:305–312, 1984

Evans DL: Recurrent instability of the ankle: a method of surgical treatment. Proc R Soc Med 46:343–344, 1953

Evans GA, Hardcastle P, Frenyo AD: Acute rupture of the lateral ligament of the ankle: to suture or not to suture? J Bone Joint Surg Br 66:209–212, 1984

Ferkel RD, Karzel RP, Del Pizzo W, et al: Arthroscopic treatment of anterolateral impingement of the ankle. Am J Sports Med 19:440–446, 1991

Ferkel RD, Scranton, PE: Current concepts review: arthroscopy of the ankle and foot. J Bone Joint Surg Am 75:1233–1242, 1993

Flick AB, Gould N: Osteochondritis dissecans of the talus (transchondral fractures of the talus): review of the literature and new surgical approach for medial dome lesions. Foot Ankle 5:165–185, 1985

Freeman MAR: Treatment of ruptures of the lateral ligaments of the ankle. J Bone Joint Surg Br 47:661–668, 1965

Freeman MAR, Dean MRE, Hanham IWF: The etiology and prevention of functional instability of the foot. J Bone Joint Surg Br 47:678–685, 1965

Garrick JG: When can I . . . ? A practical approach to the rehabilitation, illustrated by treatment of an ankle injury. Am J Sports Med 9:67–68, 1981

Gould N, Seligson D, Gassman J: Early and late repair of lateral ligaments of the ankle. Foot Ankle 1:84–89, 1980

Grace DL: Lateral ankle ligament injuries: inversion and anterior stress radiography. Clin Orthop 183:153–159, 1984

Greene TA, Hillman SK: Comparison of support provided by a semirigid orthosis and adhesive ankle taping before, during, and after exercise. Am J Sports Med 18:498–506, 1990

Hamilton WG: Foot and ankle injuries in dancers. In: Mann RA, Coughlin MJ (eds): Surgery of the Foot and Ankle, pp 1241–1277. St. Louis, Mosby, 1993

Hamilton WG: Stonosing tenosynovitis of the flexor hallucis longus tendon and posterior impingement upon the os trigonum in ballet dancers. Foot Ankle 3:74–80, 1982

Hardaker WT: Foot and ankle injuries in classical ballet dancers. Orthop Clin North AM 20:621–627, 1989

Hardaker WT, Margello S, Goldner JL: Foot and ankle injuries in theatrical dancers. Foot Ankle 6:59–69, 1985

Harper MC: Posterior instability of the talus: an anatomic evaluation. Foot Ankle 10:36, 1989

Harper MC, Keller TS: A radiographic evaluation of the tibiofibular syndesmosis. Foot Ankle 10:156–160, 1989

Hedrick MR, McBryde AM: Posterior ankle impingement. Foot Ankle 15:2–8, 1994

Heilman AE, Braly WG, Bishop JO, et al: An anatomic study of subtalar instability. Foot Ankle 10:224–228, 1990

Hontas MJ, Haddad RJ, Schlesinger, LC: Conditions of the talus in the runner. Am J Sports Med 14:486–490,1986

Hopkinson WJ, St. Pierre P, Ryan JB, et al: Syndesmosis sprains of the ankle. Foot Ankle 10:325–330, 1990

Howse AJG: Posterior block of the ankle joint in dancers. Foot Ankle 3:81–84, 1982

Jackson DW, Ashley RL, Powell JW: Ankle sprains in young athletes: relation of severeity and disability. Clin Orthop 101:201–215, 1974

Joy G, Patzakis MJ, Harvey JP Jr: Precise evaluation of the reduction of severe ankle fractures. J Bone Joint Surg Am 56:979, 1974

Kannus P, Renstrom P: Current concepts review; treatment for acute tears of the lateral ligaments of the ankle: operation, cast, or early controlled mobilization. J Bone Joint Surg Am 73:305–312, 1991

Kaye RA: Stabilization of ankle syndesmosis injuries with a syndesmosis screw. Foot Ankle 9:290–293, 1989

Kleiger B: Foot and ankle injuries in dancers. In: Norman A (ed): Radiology Diagnosis Imaging Intervention, Vol 5, pp 1–8. Philadelphia, Lippincott, 1988

Larsen E: Experimental instability of the ankle: a radiographic investigation. Clin Orthop 204:193–200, 1985

Lauge-Hansen N: Fractures of the ankle. II. Combined experimental surgical and experimental-roentgenologic investigations. Arch Surg 60:957, 1950

Laurin CA, Ouellet R, St. Jacques R: Talar and subtalar tilt: an experimental investigation. Can J Surg 11:270–279, 1968

Lian GJ, Marder RM: Open treatment of medial talar dome lesions. Presented at American Orthopaedic Foot and Ankle Society Meeting, Coeur D'Alene, ID, July 1994

Lofvenberg R, Karrholm J, Sundelin G, et al: Prolonged reaction time in patients with chronic lateral instability of the ankle. Am J Sports Med 23:414–417,1995

Loomer R, Fisher C, Lloyd-Smith R, et al: Osteochrondral lesions of the talus. Am J Sports Med 21:13–19, 1993

Martin DF, Baker CL, Curl WW, et al: Operative ankle arthroscopy: long-term followup. Am J Sports Med 17:16–23, 1989

Meislin RJ, Rose DJ, Parisien JS, Springer S: Arthroscopic treatment of synovial impingement of the ankle. Am J Sports Med 21:186–189, 1993

Moller-Larsen F, Wethelunc JO, Jurik AG, et al: Comparison of three different treatments for ruptured lateral ankle ligaments. Acta Orthop Scand 59:564–566, 1988

Mukherjee SK, Young AB: Dome fracture of the talus: a report of ten cases. J Bone Joint Surg Br 55:319–326, 1973

Muller ME, Allgower M, Schneider R, Willenegger H: Manual of Internal Fixation, 2nd ed. New York, Springer-Verlag, 1979

Naumetz VA, Schweigel JF: Osteocartilagenous lesions of the talar dome. J Trauma 20:924–927, 1980

Nitz AJ, Dobner JJ, Kersey: Nerve injury and grades II and III ankle sprains. Am J Sports Med 13:177–182, 1985

Nyska M, Amir H, Porath A, et al: Radiological assessment of a modified anterior drawer test of the ankle. Foot Ankle 13:400–403, 1992

O'Donoghue D: Impingement exostoses of the talus and tibia. J Bone Joint Surg Am 39:835, 1957

Ottaviani RA, Ashton-Miller JA, Kothari SU, et al: Basketball shoe height and the maximal muscular resistance to applied ankle inversion and eversion moments. Am J Sports Med 23:418–423, 1995

Parisien JS: Arthroscopic treatment of osteochondral lesions of the talus. Am J Sports Med 14:211–217, 1986

Parsien JS, Vangsness T: Operative anthroscopy of the ankle: three years' experience. Clin Orthop 199:46–53, 1985

Paulos LE, Johnson Cl, Noyes FR: Posterior compartment fractures of the ankle: a commonly missed athletic injury. Am J Sports Med 11:439–443, 1983

Pettine KA, Morrey BF: Osteochrondral fractures of the talus: a long-term follow-up. J Bone Joint Surg Br 69:89–92, 1987

Pritsch M, Horoshovski H, Farine I: Arthroscopic treatment of osteochrondral lesions of the talus. J Bone Surg Am 68:862–864, 1986

Quirk R: Talar compression syndrome in dancers. Foot Ankle 3:65–68, 1982

Rasmussen O: Stability of the ankle joint: analysis of the function and traumatology of the ankle ligaments. Acta Orthop Scand Suppl 211, 1985

Renstrom P, Wertz M, Incavo S, Pope M, Ostgaard HC, Arms S, Haugh L: Strain in the lateral ligaments of the ankle. Foot Ankle 9:59–63, 1988

Rijke AM, Jones B, Vierhout PA: Injury to the lateral ankle ligaments of athletes: a posttraumatic followup. Am J Sports Med 16:256–259, 1988

Rovere GD, Clarke TJ, Yates CS, et al: Retrospective comparison of taping and ankle stabilizers in preventing ankle injuries. Am J Sports Med 16:228–233, 1988

Schaffer JJ, Manoli A II: The antiglide plate for distal fibular fixation: a biomechanical comparison with fixation with a lateral plate. J Bone Joint Surg Am 69:596–604, 1987

Scharling M: Osteochondritis dissecans of the talus. Acta Orthop Scand 49:89–94, 1978

Singer KM, Jones DC: Ligament injuries of the ankle and foot. In: The Lower Extremity and Spine in Sports Medicine, Vol 1, pp 475–497. St. Louis, Mosby, 1986

Taga I, Shino K, Inoue M, et al: Articular cartilage lesions in ankles with lateral ligament injury: an arthroscopic study. Am J Sports Med 21:120–127, 1993

Taylor DC, Englehardt, DL, Bassett FH: Syndesmosis sprains of the ankle: the influence of heterotopic ossification. Am J Sports Med 20:146–150, 1992

Thompson JP, Loomer RL: Osteochrondral lesions of the talus in a sports medicine clinic: a new radiographic technique and surgical approach. Am J Sports Med 12:460–463, 1984

Van Buecken K, Barrack RL, Alexander AH, Ertl JP: Arthroscopic treatment of transchondral talar dome fractures. Am J Sports Med 17:350–356, 1989

Veazey BL, Heckman JD, Galindo MJ, McGanity PLJ: Excision of ununited fracture of the posterior process of the talus: a treatment for chornic posterior ankle pain. Foot Ankle 13:453–457, 1992

Watson-Jones R: Fractures and Joint Injuries, Vol 2, 4th ed, pp 821–823. Edinburgh, Livingstone, 1955

Weber MJ: Ankle fractures and dislocations. In: Chapman MW (ed). Operative Orthopaedics, 2nd ed. Philadelphia, Lippincott, 1993

Wredmark T, Carlstedt CA, Bauer H, Saartok T: Os trigonum syndrome: a clinical entity in ballet dancers. Foot Ankle 11:404–406, 1991

Yablon IG, Heller FG, Shouse L: The key role of the lateral malleolus in displaced fractures of the ankle. J Bone Joint Surg Am 59:169, 1977

Yvars MF: Osteochondral fractures of the dome of the talus. Clin Orthop 114:185–191, 1976

Zeegers AV, vanderWerken C: Rupture of the deltoid ligament in ankle fracture: should it be repaired? Injury 20:39–41, 1989

2
Hindfoot

Heel Pain

The heel refers to the calcaneus and the tissues that attach to and surround it. There are a variety of acute and chronic conditions and injuries in this anatomic region that commonly occur in athletes and have the potential to impair performance. These entities can usually be diagnosed by a direct history combined with careful examination. Knowledge of the anatomy of the heel and the pathologies usually involved, together with the history, guide the physical examination. For the purposes of diagnosis and treatment, it is useful to classify heel pain anatomically into posterior and subcalcaneal heel pain.

Anatomy

The calcaneus is irregularly shaped with thin cortical walls and an inner structure of cancellous bone arranged along lines of compression and tensile stress. The posterior half of the calcaneus is extraarticular, and the anterosuperior half articulates with the talus. The anterior portion has an articulation with the cuboid.

The posterior tuberosity of the calcaneus has a narrow apex and broad base (Sarrafian, 1983). At the junction between the posterior and superior surfaces is a variably shaped prominence, the superior calcaneal prominence (Angermann, 1990; Fiamengo et al., 1982; Jahss and Koy, 1983; Stephens, 1994).

Inferior to this point, at about the midpoint of the tuberosity's posterior surface, is the attachment of the Achilles tendon. The tendon has a broad insertion with bands attaching across the width of the bone. The retrocalcaneal bursa is a horseshoe-shaped synovial sac that rests between the Achilles tendon and the superior half of the posterior tuberosity, acting to protect the tendon from frictional shearing against the bone (Frey et al., 1992). The deep surface of the bursa is a fibrocartilaginous layer on the posterior calcaneal wall. The superficial surface is contiguous with the Achilles epitenon.

The Achilles tendon anchors the gastrocnemius and soleus muscles to the calcaneus (Allenmark, 1992; Clain and Baxter, 1992; Clancy et al., 1976). This large tendon has a surrounding peritenon but no true synovial sheath (Krist et al., 1987). Between the tendon and skin is a superficial adventitial bursa that can form in response to local irritation (Clain and Baxter, 1992; Smart et al., 1980).

The inferior surface contains the medial calcaneal tuberosity, from which originates the abductor hallucis and flexor digitorum brevis muscles and the plantar fascia (Karr, 1994; Sarrafian, 1983; Warren, 1990). An anterior projection of bone, a so-called heel spur, can occur in the origin of the flexor digitorum brevis muscle (Forman & Green, 1990). More laterally, at the junction of the inferior and lateral calcaneal surfaces, is the much smaller lateral tuberosity, from which originates the aductor digiti quinti muscle (Sohepsis et al., 1991).

The plantar aponeurosis, or plantar fascia, arises from the superficial portion of the medial calcaneal tuberosity. It is a thick structure at its origin, gradually thinning as it passes distally along the subcutaneous border of the foot (Kwong et al., 1988). It inserts into the proximal phalanges of the lesser toes, the sesamoids of the great toe metatarsophalangeal (MTP), and the skin of the ball of the foot (Kitaoka et al., 1994).

The posterior tibial nerve branches at the level of the medial malleolus to form the medial and lateral plantar nerves and the medial calcaneal nerve. The calcaneal branch passes posteriorly and inferiorly, becoming superficial and providing innervation for the skin of the heel.

The medial and lateral plantar nerves course deep to the abductor hallucis muscle. The first branch of the lateral plantar nerve runs from medial to lateral just distal to the medial calcaneal tuberosity, passing between the abductor hallucis and the deeper quadratus plantae (Baxter and Thigpen, 1984; Henricson and Westlin, 1984). It provides motor fibers to the abductor digiti quinti and sensory innervation for the plantar fascia and calcaneal periosteum (Schon et al., 1993).

The heel pad is unique in its shock-absorbing function. It is composed of dense strands of elastic fibrous tissue that form septa shaped like cones and circles (Jahss et al., 1992; Miller, 1982). These septa enclose closely packed fat cells and and provide a cushion to absorb the force of heel strike. The heel pad may become less elastic in patients with chronic heel pain (Prichasuk, 1994). The plantar skin also has a high resistance to abrasion (Robbins, 1994).

Posterior Heel Pain

The multiple causes of posterior heel pain can be separated anatomically into pain that occurs along the Achilles tendon, in the interval between the calcaneus and the Achilles tendon, and pain at the level of the Achilles insertion.

Achilles tendonitis can be caused by degeneration within the substance of the tendon due to inflammation of the paratenon or by calcareous deposits in the substance of the tendon (elen et al., 1989). Palpation between the calcaneus and the Achilles tendon elicits pain due to retrocalcaneal bursitis. Tenderness along one of the ridges of the tuberosity medially or laterally, or directly posterior at the level of the tendon insertion, is an insertional tendonitis. Haglund syndrome is a combination of insertional tendonitis, a large superior calcaneal tuberosity, and retrocalcaneal and superficial adventitial bursitis. Sever's syndrome is the usual cause of heel pain in children and adolescents.

Insertional Tendonitis of Achilles Tendon and Haglund Syndrome

Athletes with insertional tendonitis have a presentation similar to that of patients with retrocalcaneal bursitis and Haglunds syndrome. If fact, it may be difficult to differentiate between these problems. Fortunately, the nonoperative and operative treatments of these conditions are similar. Athletes with insertional tendonitis have pain at the midpoint of the posterior tuberosity where the tendon inserts.

Injury is caused by strain on the tendon's insertion that results in degeneration and scarring of the normal fibrous tissue in the tendon and the paratenon. There may be thickening of the tendon, posterior heel, or the ridges on either side. There also may be changes in the bone, including cyst formation and heterotopic ossification.

Pain in the heel, an enlarged superior prominence of the calcaneal tuberosity, and swelling with a soft tissue prominence posteriorly comprise Haglund syndrome. The interposed retrocalcaneal bursa protects the Achilles tendon from frictional attrition by the superior calcaneal tuberosity during dorsiflexion. When this bony prominence is enlarged or when the shoe rubs against the heel, the bursa can become irritated and lead to retrocalcaneal bursitis (Angermann, 1990; Stephens, 1994).

Further irritation causes changes in the tissue surrounding the Achilles tendon, leading to adventitial bursitis and more soft tissue swelling and thickening. The resulting posterior prominence of the heel is due to the soft tissue swelling associated with the adventitial bursitis and a bony prominence from the superior angle of the calcaneus that presses posteriorly. This prominence is termed a pump bump because the counter of the shoe is a factor in its development (Clain and Baxter, 1992; Stephens, 1994).

Physical Examination

Athletes with insertional tendonitis usually have a normal appearing heel, whereas those with Haglund syndrome have an obvious posterior prominence. The prominence may appear larger along one side, or it may be symmetric. The bump is usually tender, and the overlying skin may be erythematous because of the rubbing against the counter of the shoe. With Haglund syndrome, palpation of the Achilles insertion or the retrocalcaneal bursa reveals tenderness.

Radiography

The lateral radiograph shows the posterior calcaneal prominence to be a combination of bone and a soft tissue shadow (Fig. 2.1).

Often the soft tissue component is larger than expected from physical examination results. Attempts to quantitate the severity of the prominence of the superior calcaneal tuberosity include determination of the posterior calcaneal angle and the parallel pitch lines (Heneghan and Parlor, 1983).

The posterior calcaneal angle is measured by drawing a line along the inferior surface of the calcaneus defined by the medial calcaneal tubercle and the inferior margin of the calcaneocuboid articulation. A second line is drawn along the posterior surface of the calcaneus defined by the tuberosity for the Achilles tendon attachment at the midpoint of the bone and the upper point of the superior tubercle. The angle between these lines is the posterior calcaneal angle. If the angle is more than 75 degrees, it is considered to be pathologic (Fowler and Philip, 1945).

Another radiographic measurement is the parallel pitch. To construct this, a reference line is drawn along the inferior margin of the calcaneus as for the posterior calcaneal angle. A second line, drawn parallel to this line, passes through the most superior point of the posterior facet. If the superior prominence of the tuberosity lies above this second line, it is considered to be enlarged (Pavlov et al., 1982).

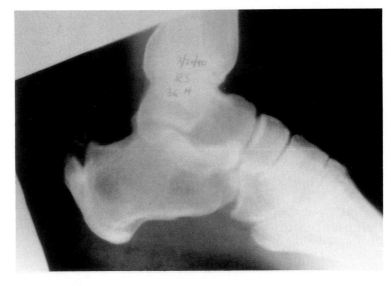

FIGURE 2.1. Haglund's deformity, retrocalcaneal bursitis, and calcific tendinitis of the Achilles tendon. (See Fig. 2.5.)

Nonoperative Treatment

The initial treatment of insertional Achilles tendonitis and Haglund syndrome are the same as for proximal Achilles tendonitis. It consists in activity restriction, oral antiinflammatory medication, heel lifts, and a gradual rehabilitation program of stretching and strengthening exercises. The pump bump is treated by modifying shoewear to relieve pressure on the prominence. Recreational shoes whose counter does not contact the pump bump should be worn. If the athletic shoe or boot can be similarly altered, it may be the only treatment required. It is sometimes possible to punch out areas of pressure (e.g., in a ski boot). Foam pads that ring the prominence may also alleviate pressure.

Operative Treatment

The surgical treatments for insertional tendonitis, retrocalcaneal bursitis, and Haglund syndrome are essentially the same. When treating these conditions, the retrocalcaneal bursa is excised and the superior prominence of the tuberosity removed, decompressing the area deep to the distal Achilles tendon (Fig. 2.2). (Sili, 1994) It is also important to remove any painful heterotopic ossification

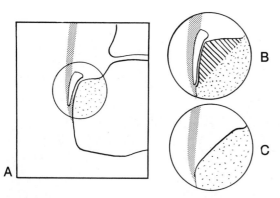

FIGURE 2.2. Haglund's deformity and retrocalcaneal bursitis. (A) Achilles tendon insertion into the calcaneus with the retrocalcaneal bursa between the tendon and the superior calcaneal tuberosity. (B) Segment of the superior calcaneal tuberosity to be removed (cross-hatching). (C) After excision of the segment of superior calcaneal tuberosity and retrocalcaneal bursa.

and the bony ridge on the end of the calcaneus if it has been identified as painful (Angermann, 1990; Stephens, 1994).

Most athletes can identify one side or the other as the site of greater pain. This point is important to determine because it has implications about the surgical approach. Because the leg rotates externally the lateral side is accessible with the patient prone, but the medial side is obscured. Athletes whose symptoms are predominant on the lateral side or directly posterior and those who have bilateral involvement should be treated in the prone position. If the pain is mostly posteromedial, the supine position is used with a bump placed under the opposite hip.

Surgical Decompression

Technique

1. Appropriate anesthesia and a thigh tourniquet are used. The patient is positioned according to the guidelines mentioned above. A 5 cm longitudinal incision is made along the side of the Achilles tendon from the level of the inferior border of the calcaneus proximally.
2. In the proximal wound, the fat pad is separated from the Achilles tendon. This interval is followed distally until the retrocalcaneal bursa is entered. The incision continues inferiorly through the bursa, just in front of the tendon, until the level of its insertion is reached (Fig. 2.3).
3. The scalpel is used to slightly elevate the fibers of insertion and calcaneal periosteum where they merge on the edge of the calcaneus. Subperiosteal elevation reveals the underlying bone for a short distance (3–5 mm).
4. The superior prominence of the tuberosity is generously removed with an osteotome (Figs. 2.4, 2.5), being careful to not plunge through the skin on the opposite side. The osteotome and rongeurs contour the bone so no sharp edges remain.
5. The retrocalcaneal bursa is removed using a rongeur and scalpel.
6. Any preoperative tenderness along the prominence of the exposed edge of the calcaneus is an indication for its removal.

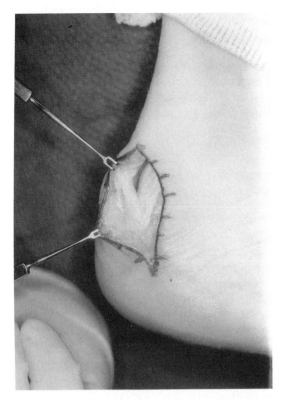 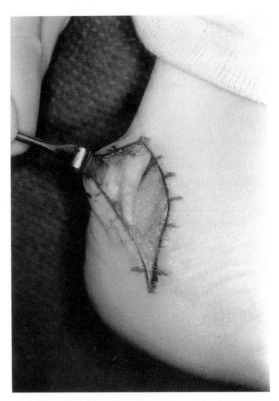

FIGURE 2.3. Haglund's deformity and retrocalcaneal bursitis. An incision is made along the lateral edge of the heel parallel to the Achilles tendon. The tendon is shown inserting into the calcaneal tuberosity with the retrocalcaneal space displayed.

FIGURE 2.4 Haglund's deformity and retrocalcaneal bursitis. The superior segment of the posterior calcaneal tuberosity has been excised, leaving a surface of cancellous bone exposed. The Achilles tendon is seen posterior to this point.

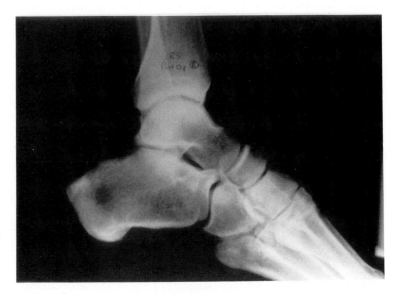

FIGURE 2.5. Haglund's deformity and retrocalcaneal bursitis. The superior calcaneal tuberosity and calcified segment of Achilles tendon have been excised. (See Fig. 2.1.)

The periosteum and Achilles tendon, which had been elevated, are preserved to be used for closing over this wound when the operationis completed. If there is tenderness on both sides, the opposite edge can often be satisfactorily taken down through the same incision. An alternative is to roll the table back and make a second incision along the opposite side of the Achilles tendon. This maneuver risks devascularizing the enclosed segment of the distal skin, but in practice it is not a problem, provided the incisions are made anterior to the tendon on both sides, leaving an adequate bridge of skin.

7. Finally, if there is heteotopic ossification within the distal tendon or at the site of insertion, it is removed. Removal is done from the deep side of the tendon, with a small retractor aiding in visualization. A longitudinal incision is made in the tendon, and the extra bone is excised or removed with a rongeur, care being taken not to disrupt fibers of the Achilles tendon.

8. During closure it is important to repair the elevated calcaneal periosteum to the edge of the Achilles tendon with interrupted stitches of 0 absorbable suture. The subcutaneous and skin layers are then closed in layers, and a short leg cast is applied.

Postoperative Management. The patient is kept non-weight-bearing for 10 to 14 days, at which time the skin sutures are removed. If disruption of the Achilles attachment was deemed to be small and the repair of the periosteum to the edge of the tendon satisfactory, the patient is allowed to begin partial weight-bearing in a regular shoe. Walking in a regular shoe is the extent of activity until 8 weeks after surgery, at which time all activities are allowed to tolerance.

If the Achilles attachment was significantly elevated to remove heterotopic calcification or to expose the posterior calcaneal edges, a short-leg walking cast is used until 6 weeks after surgery. Physical therapy and unrestricted weight-bearing are then started, and 10 weeks after surgery full return to athletic activities is allowed.

Sever's Syndrome (Calcaneal Apophysitis)

Sever's syndrome is the most common cause of heel pain in children and adolescents (Micheli and Ireland, 1987). It is an overuse injury of the calcaneal apophysis often seen in adolescent athletes. It is similar to, and may coexist with, Osgood-Schlatter syndrome.

Clinical Presentation

According to a review by Micheli and Ireland (1987), the average age of presentation for boys and girls with Sever's syndrome is approximately 11 years. The children experienced pain with a variety of athletic activities, and more than half were unable to participate because of pain (Micheli and Ireland, 1987).

Patients have tenderness to compression of the tuberosity of the calcaneus (Gregg and Das, 1982; Griffin, 1994). They may also have tightness of the heel cord, or Achilles tendon (Micheli and Ireland, 1987).

Radiography

The calcaneal apophysis is a secondary ossification center that appears at age 9 years and completely fuses by age 16 years (Micheli and Ireland, 1987). The radiographic appearance of the apophysis in normal individuals shows irregularities and sclerosis, and there is no difference in patients with Sever syndrome (Gregg and Das, 1982).

Treatment

The goal of treatment is to put the heel at rest, which is accomplished by restricting athletic activities for 2 to 4 weeks along with use of a heel lift. If symptoms persist, use of a walking cast may provide relief. Stretching exercises aimed at heel cord tightness are instituted (Griffin, 1994; Micheli and Ireland, 1987). There is no need for oral antiinflammatory medication or steroid injection. Micheli and Ireland (1987) found complete resolution with nonoperative treatment by an average of 2 months.

Subcalcaneal Heel Pain

Plantar heel pain is one of the most common problems encountered by foot specialists. Although the etiology of the pain is poorly understood, treatment is usually successful. The most common pattern is associated with maximal tenderness at the anteromedial side of the heel pad, defined as plantar fasciitis. Much less common is pain due to a calcaneal stress fracture or that secondary to poor padding in the soft tissue of the heel.

Plantar Fasciitis

Plantar fasciitis is thought to be caused by a traction injury at the origin of the plantar fascia on the medial calcaneal tubercle. It rarely occurs with an acute, identifiable injury but usually develops insidiously. With continued activity, chronic inflammation and symptoms develop.

Plantar fasciitis is the most common cause of heel pain, and heel pain is the most common problem seen in foot clinics (Davis et al., 1994). This problem is well recognized in runners and dancers and has been reported in a wide variety of athletes who are involved in running activities (Henricson and Westlin, 1984; Kwong et al., 1988; Leach et al., 1984).

Etiology

Excessive stress causes microtears in the fascia at the fascia–bone interface that coalesce with continued loading, forming a symptomatic mass (Chandler and Kibler, 1993). Support for this theory comes from surgical pathologic specimens that have identified mucoid degeneration, inflammation, and chronic granulomatous tissue in the plantar fascia (Leach et al., 1983; Leach et al., 1986; Snider et al., 1983).

Neuritis has also been proposed as a cause of this pain. The medial calcaneal nerve has been implicated, as has the first branch of the lateral plantar nerve, the nerve to the abductor digiti quinti (Baxter and Thigpen, 1984; Schon et al., 1993). It is possible that the neuritis is a secondary phenomenon, with inflammation developing from positioning adjacent to the plantar fascia origin.

The role of the plantar traction spur at the medial calcaneal tubercle is unclear (Schepsis et al., 1991). This spur lies deep to the plantar fascia at the level of the origin of the flexor digitorum brevis. The lay population and many physicians refer to plantar fascia pain as "heel spur" pain, believing the spur to be the cause of the pain. Certainly, many athletes describe a sensation of "walking on a sharp piece of bone sticking into the heel." There may be a higher incidence of radiographically evident heel spurs in patients with plantar fasciitis than in the general population (Tanz, 1963). However, a significant number of patients with pain have no evidence of a heel spur (Davis et al., 1994; Kwong et al., 1988; Rubin and Witten, 1963).

Clinical Presentation

The clinical description of pain is generally characteristic. Most athletes note the gradual onset of pain in the heel that originally is associated with activity and relieved by rest. As the problem progresses, the pain is worse with the first few steps each morning or when arising from prolonged sitting. It may then improve only to return later in the day. Finally, running and jumping are affected, limiting performance, with pain becoming nearly constant. Often athletes have had the pain for many months before seeking medical attention.

Examination

The characteristic finding is tenderness at the anteromedial border of the heel pad. The distal plantar fascia may also be tender and should be evaluated for defects or nodules. Tenderness along the medial or lateral walls of the calcaneus is potentially pain due to a stress fracture; posterior tenderness suggests Achilles tendonitis. The posterior tibial nerve is percussed to exclude tarsal tunnel syndrome as a cause of the pain.

Radiography

The lateral radiograph of the foot may reveal a plantar traction spur, which is of questionable importance (Davis et al., 1994; Rubin and Witen, 1993; Schepsis et al., 1991; Williams, 1987). Spurs are found frequently in the general population, occurring in asymptomatic people, and increasing with age, they may have no direct relation to heel pain (Wall et al., 1993).

In cases of diagnostic uncertainty, a technetium bone scan may be helpful. Early blood pool images correlate with active inflammation and may identify plantar fasciitis, differentiating it from a calcaneal stress fracture (Vasavada, et al., 1984). The delayed images may show tracer uptake along the inferior border of the calcaneus, indicating either periostitis or an inflammatory abnormality in the area (Sewell et al., 1980). In one study, delayed images were positive in about 60% of patients with plantar fasciitis with no false positive results (Williams et al., 1987).

Ultrasonography has been reported to identify thickening in the plantar fascia of patients with a known clinical diagnosis (Wall et al., 1993). It identifies areas of focal and diffuse hypoechogenicity, which reflect inflammation. Similar findings of plantar fascia thickening and increased intrasubstance signal intensity, consistent with inflammation, have been seen with magnetic resonance imaging (MRI) (Berkowitz et al., 1991).

Nonoperative Treatment

For most patients nonoperative treatment is satisfactory (Wolgin et al., 1994). Most studies indicate that 5% of patients, however, ultimately require surgery (Bordelon, 1993; McBryde, 1984).

Three treatment modalities form the basis of the initial treatment: an oral nonsteroidal antiinflammatory drug (NSAID), steroid injection, and taping of the arch. If the athlete has an early or mild case or is in the middle of the athletic season and cannot take time off, injection and taping can be deferred. In this case, a course of antiinflammatory medication is given along with a soft viscoelastic heel pad placed in the shoe to improve cushioning. Each day after athletic activity the heel and arch are treated with ice massage for 20 to 30 minutes.

If the athlete has significant symptoms and the training program allows it, the three modalities are used simultaneously. Steroid injection and arch taping are performed initially with an oral NSAID prescribed for 10 to 14 days. The tape is left in place for 7 days. The athlete is instructed to eliminate all but essential activities for 10 days. Most patients have significant improvement or complete relief by the time the tape is removed. If symptoms persist, the NSAID is continued for 1 month, at which point a second cortisone injection is administered.

A number of other nonoperative modalities have been recommended for the treatment of plantar fasciitis. Hard functional orthotics are sometimes prescribed but often are uncomfortable at the site of tenderness. A longitudinal arch support with medial posting may be helpful in the patient with significant pronation posture, which can increase stress on the plantar fascia.

Stretching exercises for the Achilles tendon and bent-knee stretches for the plantar fascia are helpful. Ultrasound and iontophoresis are sometimes prescribed. Dorsiflexion night splints have been shown to be an effective treatment if worn regularly for 3 to 4 months (Wapner and Sharkey, 1991). Night splints appear to work by keeping the plantar fascia on stretch, preventing the nocturnal contracture that is responsible for pain on arising in the morning. For severe symptoms a short-leg cast for 3 to 4 weeks may be attempted.

Steroid Injection and Arch Taping

1. A 5 ml syringe is filled with a mixture of 1% lidocaine and 0.5% bupivacaine (Marcaine), each without epinephrine. A 3 ml syringe is filled with 1 ml of triamcinolone (Kenalog) 40 mg/ml. A 25 gauge 1.5 inch needle is attached to the larger syringe.
2. The patient is supine on the examining table. The site of maximum tenderness is located at the anteromedial border of the heel pad. After preparing the skin with antiseptic solution, the skin is treated with a spray of ethyl chloride for 3 to 5 seconds for anesthesia.
3. The needle of the local anesthetic syringe is inserted through the skin at this point

FIGURE 2.6. Origin of plantar fascia. (A) The plantar fascia originates from the medial calcaneal tuberosity, just superficial to a traction spur, if present. (B) Site of surgical division of the plantar fascia for treating chronic plantar fasciitis.

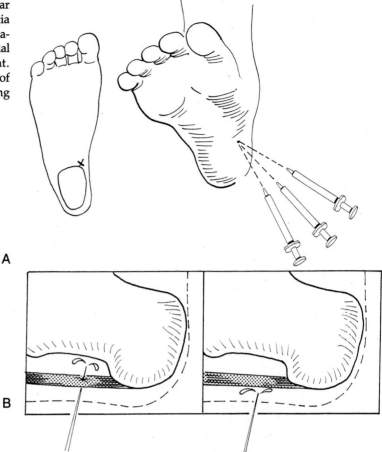

A

B

(Fig. 2.6). As the needle is advanced, the local anesthetic is slowly injected. Continuing deeper, the thick plantar fascia is encountered as slight resistance, and the needle is passed through it.

4. First, a small amount of the local anesthetic is injected deep to the fascia (approximately 0.5 ml) (Fig. 2.7). The needle is slowly withdrawn until it is just superficial to the fascia, and a similar small amount of local anesthetic is injected. The angle of the syringe is then changed so the needle is directed slightly more laterally, and again it is advanced through the fascia. Another small amount of local is deposited in this location, the needle withdrawn until it is again superficial to the fascia more laterally, and another injection is given. This step is repeated three or four times, spreading the local anesthetic along the width of the plantar fascia both deep and superficial to it. A small amount of the anesthetic (0.5–1.0 ml) should be left in the syringe.

5. The needle is left in place, with care taken so that it is either deep or superficial to, but not within, the fascia. This syringe is then removed from the needle, and the smaller syringe containing the cortisone is attached.

6. The movement of the needle is repeated so the steroid is spread into the same areas into which the anesthetic had been injected (Fig. 2.7). Only 0.1 to 0.2 ml of steroid is injected at each point. *It is important not to inject steroid into the substance of the plantar fascia, as it can cause necrosis and lead to rupture.*

7. The small syringe is then removed, again leaving the needle in place. The larger

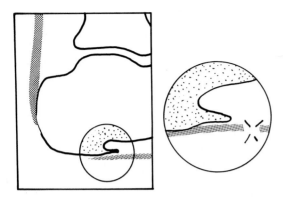

FIGURE 2.7. Steroid injection for plantar fasciitis. The injection is given at the anteromedial border of the heel pad. The needle is passed several times, changing its angle to spread the steroid along the width of the fascia. Injection is deep and superficial to the fascia but not into the substance of the fascia.

syringe is replaced on the needle, and as the needle is withdrawn through the skin the remaining local anesthetic is injected. This step ensures that no steroid is inadvertently deposited in the subcutaneous fat or the skin, where it could induce fat necrosis, skin dimpling, or depigmentation. The area of the injection is then massaged for 20 to 30 seconds to spread the injected medication around.

8. Arch taping is then performed. Tincture of benzoin is applied as a liquid or spray to the ball of the foot, the arch, and behind the heel. This substance protects the skin and helps the tape to stick. Three strips of 1 inch adhesive tape are placed transversely across the ball of the foot to act as an anchoring base.

9. A 12 inch long piece of tape is placed against the back of the heel at the level of the Achilles insertion. One length of this tape runs along the medial side of the heel, under the arch, and onto the lateral side of the tape on the ball of the foot. The other length of this tape runs over the lateral side of the heel, crossing over its other end in the arch and attaching to the medial side of the transverse tape on the ball of the foot. This taping is repeated with another strand of tape.

10. Three more transverse strands of tape are placed across the ball of the foot, locking

the two long loops on both sides between the two layers and anchoring them to the forefoot. The tape is covered with a layer of Coban, which helps prevent unraveling.

Operative Treatment

For those athletes who have failed an adequate course of nonoperative treatment, surgery is considered. Spontaneous rupture of the plantar fascia in patients with proceeding symptoms of plantar fasciitis has been shown to cure the symptoms after 4 weeks. (Ahlstrom et al., 1988; Herrick and Herrick, 1983). Lutter (1986) recommended that surgery be deferred until at least 12 months from the start of treatment. Other reports suggest that athletes who have persistent pain after 5 to 7 months can be treated operatively (Leach et al., 1986; Snider et al., 1983). The surgical procedures involve dividing all or part of the plantar fascia at its origin on the medial calcaneal tubercle. Some authors remove the bone spur, whereas others leave it. Excellent results are obtained in 71% to 100% of operated patients (Anderson and Foster, 1989; Kahn et al., 1985; Leach et al., 1986; Lester and Buchanan, 1984; Schepsis et al., 1991; Snider et al., 1983).

There is evidence that surgically disrupting the plantar fascia may alter the shape of the arch, causing it to lose height (Daly et al., 1992). A consequence of the loss of the plantar fascia is the development of pain on the dorsum of the midfoot in some patients (Sellman, 1994).

The technique of endoscopic plantar fascia release has been championed as a minimally invasive method for surgical treatment (Barrett and Day, 1991). There have been problems reported with this procedure, however, including division of the plantar nerves and blood vessels.

The traditional approach for plantar fascia release is through a medial longitudinal incision, although this approach does not allow direct visualization of the fascia that is to bereleased. The endoscopic technique also provides a poor view of the structures, which probably contributes to the complications associated with this procedure. A transverse plantar incison allows the entire width of the plantar fascia to be seen and prevents inadvertent damage to the underlying muscle and neurovascular structures (Kahn et al., 1985; Lewis et al., 1991).

Plantar Fascia Release. The bony spur is not removed during plantar fascia release (Fig. 2.8). The first branch of the lateral plantar nerve is necessarily decompressed by the release, but the nerve is not dissected free. The entire width of the fascia is divided.

Technique

1. The procedure is performed with the patient in the prone position. A general anesthetic or ankle block can be used, either being administered in the supine position on a gurney. The patient is then rolled onto the operating room table in the prone position. A thigh tourniquet is used with a general anesthetic, and an Esmarch tourniquet wrapped about the ankle is used with an ankle block.
2. A 5 cm transverse incision is made on the plantar aspect of the foot at the anterior edge of the heel pad, so it is located away from the weight-bearing area. The thick layer of fat is divided with the scalpel in line with the incision. A small Weitlaner retractor can be inserted to help with visualization.
3. The plantar fascia is just below the fat, and the fat is swept anteriorly and posteriorly off the fascia so it is visualized across the entire width of the foot (Fig. 2.8).
4. A no. 15 scalpel is used to divide the fascia for its entire width. Care is taken to avoid dividing the underlying muscle. The fascia retracts 4 to 5 mm after the division (Fig. 2.9).
5. After irrigating the wound, the deep fat is loosely approximated with interrupted stitches of 2-0 absorbable suture. The skin is then closed with simple interrupted stitches of 3-0 nonabsorbable suture. Care is taken so the layers line up properly when closing the skin so as to minimize the chance of a thick scar forming. A soft dressing is applied.

Postoperative Management. The patient is kept non-weight-bearing, using crutches for 3 weeks. The dressing is removed after 1 week to inspect the wound. Bathing can begin. At 3 weeks point, the skin sutures are removed, and progressive weight-bearing is allowed. A composite longitudinal arch support is then made using plastizote and PPT, which the patient wears for 3 months in both recreational and athletic shoes. Training may resume as early as 6 weeks after surgery.

Painful Heel Pad

Pain localized in the center of the heel is much less common than that found at the anteromedial border of the heel pad. Central pain is due to a lack of heel padding. Atrophy of the heel pad may be due to repetitive trauma or degenerative changes (Jahss et al., 1992; Karr, 1994; Prichasuk, 1994). These changes, in turn, lead to stress on the underlying bone, with pain due to bone contusion or periostitis.

Clinical Presentation

There may be an acute onset that follows forceful impact on the heel, such as that produced by striking the heel on a hard object or falling from a height. The pain may also develop gradually in a athlete who repeatedly irritates the undersurface of the heel and whose activity level does not allow healing to take place.

Physical examination reveals the heel pad to be tender, but the tenderness is in the center of the pad, in contrast to that seen with plantar fasciitis, which is maximal at the anteromedial edge of the heel pad. Athletes with a stress fracture may have significant pain and tenderness along the wall of the calcaneus medially and laterally. Some athletes have an atrophic heel pad, which can be unilateral or bilateral. The opposite heel should be carefully examined.

Radiography

The radiographs are characteristically unremarkable. A technetium bone scan may show mildly increased tracer uptake along the plantar surface of the calcaneus, indicating contusion or periostitis.

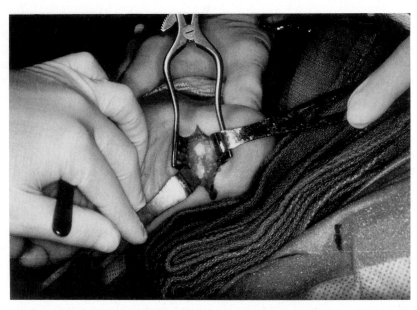

FIGURE 2.8. Surgical release for chronic plantar fasciitis. A transverse incision is made at the anterior edge of the heel pad with the plantar fascia exposed (white).

Nonoperative Treatment

This lesion is essentially a padding problem, whether there is too little in the heel itself or in the shoe. Proper shoewear must be emphasized to prevent recurrence. The training surface can be altered to a softer one, for instance asking runners to avoid concrete.

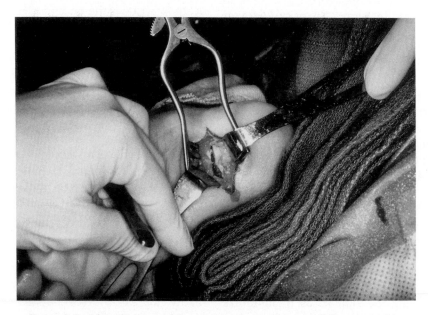

FIGURE 2.9. After division of the plantar fascia there is slight separation.

Using training shoes with thicker heel padding or adding heel pads to the shoes is usually effective and allows continued training; it can prevent recurrence in the future as well. During the acute phase limiting or avoiding activity is based on symptoms and usually results in relief.

Calcaneal Stress Fracture

Stress fracture of the calcaneus is another cause of plantar heel pain (Hullinger, 1994; Leabhart, 1959). It may result from poor intrinsic padding or inadequate shoe padding combined with extensive activity. Significant tenderness along the medial or lateral calcaneal walls is highly suggestive.

Clinical Presentation

As with other stress fractures, there may be an acute onset of pain or a gradual development of symptoms. The pain initially may be present only with high stress activities and then progressly affect weight-bearing.

On examination, tenderness about the plantar aspect of the heel is seen to be present and characteristically is found along the sides as well. Squeezing the heel can be painful if there is a stress fracture. These fractures have no accompanying swelling or ecchymosis, as is seen with an acute calcaneal fracture. There is no limitation of ankle or hindfoot motion.

Radiography

Radiographs may show a stress fracture if it has been present for at least 2 to 3 weeks. There is increased bone formation along a line in the substance of the bone, but it may not be present or may prove difficult to discriminate from the normal lines of stress in the bone. If there is uncertainty about the diagnosis, a technetium bone scan can show significantly increased isotope concentration within the bone on delayed scanning. This picture is distinguishable from that of periostitis, contusion, or the inflammation that occurs with plantar fasciitis and can produce uptake early on blood pool scans or appear on the surface of the bone.

Treatment

Treatment requires decreased in impact activities until symptoms have resolved. Substitute activities such as swimming and bicycling can be undertaken. If pain is present with weight-bearing, crutches should be used. Four to six weeks should be sufficient for successful treatment.

Tarsal Coalition

Tarsal coalition is a congenital problem that does not manifest until early adolescence or later. The coalition is a union between two of the hindfoot bones, most commonly the calcaneus and navicular or the talus and calcaneus. This union may be fibrous, cartilaginous, or bony. It is due to failure of separation of the involved bones during development (Elkus, 1986; Swiontkowski et al., 1983).

In young children the coalition between the bones is cartilaginous, which allows motion that is normal or, if restricted, is functional. During adolescence the coalition begins to ossify and may become a complete or incomplete bony bridge. As ossification proceeds, motion between bones decreases and may become entirely restricted.

When hindfoot motion is restricted, a twisting injury whose force might otherwise be dissipated through the several hindfoot joints may instead concentrate its action at the ankle, leading to an inversion sprain. Tarsal coalition has been shown to be associated with a high incidence of ankle sprains in adolescent athletes (Morgan and Crawford, 1986; Snyder et al., 1981).

Clinical Presentation

Adolescent atheletes present with the insidious onset of hindfoot pain with or without recurrent ankle sprains. Some complain of stiffness in the hindfoot. The pain is usually described as coming from the lateral side of the hindfoot and ankle.

Not only adolescents but older athletes as well may develop symptoms from a tarsal coalition. If there has been incomplete ossification of the coalition, hindfoot motion may be sufficiently satisfactory to allow normal foot function into adulthood. A twisting injury may then stretch, tear, or otherwise disrupt the coalition, causing the coalition itself to become painful. This pain is often initially diagnosed as an ankle sprain, although it is not alleviated with the usual therapies.

All patients with tarsal coalition have the key finding of absent or diminished subtalar motion. The hindfoot cannot to be everted or inverted when holding the ankle in the neutral position.

Radiography

Radiographs should be obtained, including AP, lateral, and oblique views of the foot. A calcaneonavicular coalition can usually be seen on the oblique view (Fig. 2.10). A talocalcaneal coalition usually involves the middle facet of the subtalar joint which is near the sustentaculum tali. This condition is sometimes difficult to appreciate on standard radiographic views, and Broden views or computed tomography (CT) scanning (Fig. 2.11) of the subtalar joint is necessary (Herzenberg et al., 1986).

An important finding on routine radiographs that should alert the observer to the possibility of a tarsal coalition is a dorsal beak on the neck of the talus. This beak, which represents a talonavicular traction spur, is indicative of increased stress at that joint. The presence of this beak does not indicate that arthritis or adaptive changes have occurred in the hindfoot (O'Neill and Micheli, 1989; Swiontkowski et al., 1983).

Nonoperative Treatment

Nonoperative treatment has limited benefit when treating tarsal coalition in athletes (Morgan and Crawford, 1986; O'Neill and Micheli, 1989). An initial course of immobilization in a short-leg walking cast can be tried for 3 to 6 weeks, which allows the irritation and inflammation to resolve and the child to

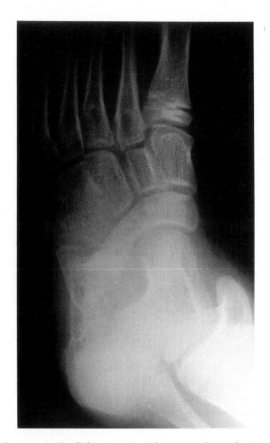

FIGURE 2.10. Calcaneonavicular tarsal coalition. Oblique radiograph of coalition involving the calcaneus and navicular.

resume athletics (Elkus, 1986; Morgan and Crawford, 1986). Should this trial be successful, taping the ankle and hindfoot or the use of an ankle brace should be encouraged if the patient wishes to continue with sports activities. In most cases when the child attains relief with nonoperative treatment, the stresses of athletics eventually cause recurrence of symptoms (Morgan and Crawford, 1986), in which case the patient is usually not satisfied with nonoperative treatment and so considers surgery.

Operative Treatment

Excellent results have been obtained with surgical excision of both calcaneonavicular and subtalar coalitions, even in the presence

FIGURE 2.11. Subtalar tarsal coalition. CT scan of tarsal coalition of
the medial subtalar joint.

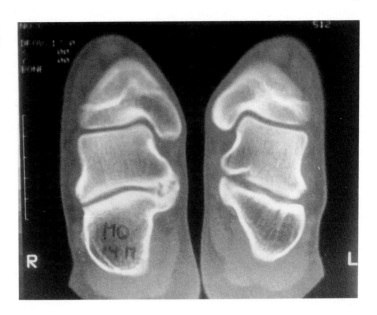

of a significant talar beak (Elkus and Crawford, 1986; Morgan 1986; O'Neill and Micheli,
1989) and should be considered the treatment
of choice in the young athlete. The alternative
surgical treatment is an arthrodesis of the
hindfoot. This operation eliminates pain but
at the expense of function, however which
negatively affects athletic performance.
Should excision of the coalition not be successful, arthrodesis can be subsequently
performed.

Subtalar coalitions involve the middle facet
and arise just above the sustentaculum tali.
They are approached through a medial hindfoot incision. Calcaneonavicular coalitions
occur in the anterior part of the sinus tarsi
and are approached laterally.

Excision of Subtalar Coalition (Medial)

Technique

1. Under tourniquet control, a 5 cm oblique
   incision is made, centered over the palpable sustentaculum tali inferior to the
   medial malleolus. The incision runs parallel to the line of the flexor tendons underneath the malleolus.
2. The tendon sheath of the flexor digitorum
   longus is opened the extent of the skin

incision. The tendon is retracted inferiorly,
protecting the neurovascular bundle.
3. The deep border of the sheath and underlying periosteum are then split in the same
   line and elevated superiorly and inferiorly
   to expose the coalition. The anterior and
   posterior extent of the coalition must be
   determined and can be marked with small
   needles to define the area of excision.
4. A small osteotome is used to cut a trape-
   zoidal segment of bone with borders 3 to 4
   mm above the coalition in the talus, 3 to 4
   mm below in the calcaneus, and anterior
   and posterior margins at the previously
   defined edges. The superior and inferior
   cuts should be oriented to converge about
   1 cm deep.
5. After removing the block of bone, further
   excision may be required to remove the
   entire coalition. It is best to do it with small
   increments of excision so the normal joint
   is not injured.
6. The joint is put through its range of motion
   to verify that the excision has been adequate. The bone edges are smoothed, and
   bone wax is applied to them.
7. The periosteum is closed with interrupted
   2-0 absorbable sutures. The flexor digitorum longus tendon is returned to its
   normal position and its sheath repaired

with a running stitch of 0 absorbable suture. After closing the skin a short-leg splint is applied.

Postoperative Management

The patient kept non-weight-bearing, with the splint worn for 10 to 14 days, at the end of which time the skin sutures are removed. The patient continues on crutches, non-weight-bearing, for 6 weeks after the surgery. Range of motion exercises are started when the sutures are removed. Return to activity usually occurs at approximately 2 to 3 months.

Excision of Calcaneonavicular Coalition (Lateral)

Technique

1. A 5 cm incision is made, centered over the sinus tarsi and running obliquely parallel to a line from the anterior border of the lateral malleolus to the tip of the fifth metatarsal styloid.
2. The flexor digitorum brevis origin lies over the sinus tarsi, and the muscle must be protected when entering the sinus. Such protection is accomplished by cutting three sides of a square around the muscle and reflecting it distally on the fourth side. Each of the cut sides is about 2 cm in length.
3. The coalition is identified, as is the calcaneocuboid joint.
4. The normal superior extent of the calcaneus and lateral extent of the navicular are defined, and the abnormal bridge between them is excised with an osteotome. The foot is put through a range of motion, and if any impingement remains in this area it is removed.
5. The bone edges are then covered with bone wax. Alternatively, the flexor digitorum brevis muscle can be reflected and inserted into the space previously occupied by the coalition, maintained by several simple stitches of 2–0 absorbable suture.
6. After closing the skin, a short-leg splint is applied.

Postoperative Management

The patient is kept non-weight-bearing for 6 weeks. After suture removal at 10 to 14 days, range-of-motion exercises are started. Activity is advanced as tolerated, after resumption of weight-bearing.

Avulsion Fractures

Anterior Process of Calcaneus Fracture

Fracture of the anterior process of the calcaneus is an avulsion injury that can be confused with an inversion ankle sprain (Fig. 2.12) (Gellman, 1954).

Anatomy

The anterior process of the calcaneus is a dorsal beak adjacent to the cuboid. It occupies the distal surface of the calcaneus, where it forms the superior edge of the calcaneocuboid joint. If prominent, it may have a small articulation with the undersurface of the talar neck (DeLee, 1993). The anterior process serves as the origin of ligaments attaching to the lateral navicular and dorsal cuboid. The inferior portion of the extensor digitorum-

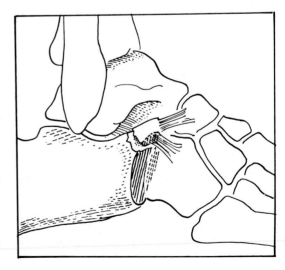

Figure 2.12. Avulsion fracture of the anterior process of the calcaneus.

brevis origin also arises from the anterior process.

Clinical Presentation

The anterior calcaneal process is fractured when the foot is forced into plantarflexion and inversion (Gellman, 1954). An ankle sprain is caused by a similar mechanism. Key to differentiating between the two injuries, either of which can cause significant swelling over the lateral ankle and foot, is the point tenderness found distal to the ankle ligaments over the lateral side of the hindfoot. Also, manipulation of the ankle into inversion is less painful than manipulation of the foot into inversion with the ankle stabilized.

Radiography

The fracture may be seen on the lateral view of the ankle if there is displacement. An oblique radiograph usually demonstrates the fracture. A radiograph with the beam directed 20 degrees superiorly and 20 degreesposteriorly has been described (DeLee, 1993). CT scanning can be performed if uncertainty exists.

Nonoperative Treatment

Fractures that are minimal or nondisplaced are best treated with immobilization in a nonweight-bearing short-leg walking cast or orthosis for 4 weeks. Motion exercises can be started after 2 weeks if symptoms allow. Protected weight-bearing is then allowed until 6 to 8 weeks after injury; and if the symptoms have resolved, activities can be advanced.

Operative Treatment

If the fracture is significantly displaced but small, it should be excised. If it is a large fragment, open reduction and internal fixation are performed.

Open Reduction and Internal Fixation

Technique

1. Under appropriate anesthesia and tourniquet control, the patient is positioned supine with a bump underneath the ipsilateral hip to improve visualization of the lateral side of the hindfoot.
2. A 5 cm oblique incision is made over the sinus tarsi, extending distally to the peroneal tendons. Care must be taken to avoid damage to the peroneal tendons and the sural nerve in the distal end of the wound.
3. The inferior edge of the extensor digitorum brevis muscle is elevated upward from the lateral side of the anterior calcaneal process, revealing the fracture. The fracture surfaces are irrigated and freshened, and the fragment is fixed into place with a provisional 0.062 inch K-wire. Fixation is then performed with a 4.0 mm cancellous screw placed from the lateral superior edge and directed posteriorly and inferiorly into the body of the calcaneus. Intraoperative radiographs are obtained to verify the reduction and screw placement.
4. After closing the wound in layers, a posterior splint is applied.

Postoperative Management. The skin sutures are removed, and a removable orthosis is applied at 14 days. Gentle motion exercises are allowed with weight-bearing after 4 weeks. Shoewear can be resumed after 6 weeks. Athletic activities should be deferred until 8 weeks after surgery.

Excision of Anterior Process of Calcaneus Fracture

Technique

1. The exposure is the same as for open reduction and internal fixation of an anterior process fracture. The fragment is sharply dissected from its ligamentous attachments. If there is a significant defect, the ligaments can be imbricated with 0 absorbable suture.
2. After closing the wound in layers a posterior splint is applied.

Postoperative Management. The skin sutures are removed at 10 to 14 days and an orthosis applied. Weight-bearing is allowed at this time. Motion, however, should be deferred until 3 to 4 weeks after the surgery. Protected weight-bearing is continued with the orthosis for an additional 3 weeks, and then activities are advanced as tolerated.

Lateral Talar Process Fracture

Fracture of the lateral process of the talus is an avulsion injury that may be confused with an ankle sprain.

Anatomy

The lateral process of the talus is a wedge-shaped prominence, extending from articulation for the fibula to the subtalar joint inferiorly (Mukerjee et al., 1974). Its greatest prominence lies between these articular surfaces, where it provides attachments for the anterior talofibular ligament, the lateral talocalcaneal ligament, and the cervical ligament.

Clinical Presentation

The injury results from a combined dorsiflexion and inversion mechanism that stresses the lateral talocalcaneal and anterior talofibular ligaments (DeLee, 1993; Hawkins, 1965; Mukherjee et al., 1974). As stress is increased, the ligaments fail or avulse the lateral process of the talus (Fig. 2.13).

The history and physical examination are similar to that for a lateral ankle sprain involving the anterior talofibular ligament. Point tenderness is located over the ligament and its talar attachment, and there is swelling and ecchymosis. Stress fracture of the lateral talar process has also been reported with the gradual onset of lateral ankle pain during sporting activities (Motto, 1993).

Radiography

The fracture can be seen on standard ankle radiographs and is best visualized on the mortise view (Fig. 2.14). If uncertainty exists, CT scanning can be confirmatory (Fig. 2.15).

Nonoperative Treatment

Prompt recognition of the fracture allows treatment to be most effective. Nondisplaced fractures are treated by immobilization in a short-leg cast for 6 weeks, with 3 weeks of

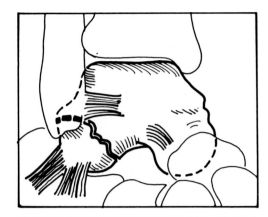

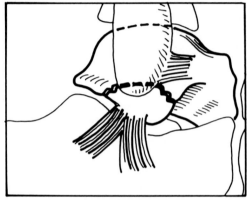

Figure 2.13. Avulsion fracture of the lateral process of the talus.

nonweight-bearing followed by 3 weeks of weight-bearing.

Operative Treatment

Displaced fractures that are of significant size should be treated with open reduction and internal fixation. Small, displaced fragments and large fragments recognized later than 2 to 3 months after injury should be treated by excision (DeLee, 1993; Hawkins, 1965; Mukherjee et al., 1974).

Open Reduction and Internal Fixation

Technique

1. A 5 cm longitudinal incision is made over the anterolateral ankle, parallel to the anterior border of the fibula and extending 1

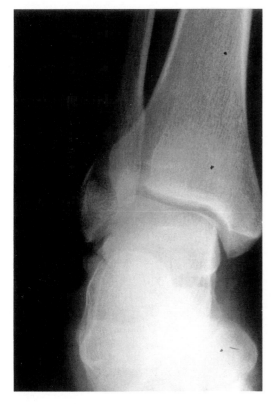

FIGURE 2.14. Avulsion fracture of the lateral process of the talus.

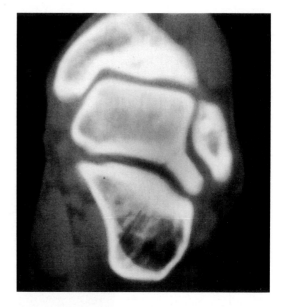

FIGURE 2.15. CT scan of a fracture of the lateral process of the talus.

cm below the tip of the fibula. The peroneal tendons are protected distally.

2. Hematoma is evacuated and the fracture anatomically reduced. A 0.062 inch K-wire can be used for provisional fixation. Fixation is achieved by one or more 4.0 mm cancellous screws inserted in the nonarticular prominence of the fragment, directed obliquely upward into the body of the talus. Intraoperative radiographs are obtained to assess the screw position and the quality of reduction (Fig. 2.16).

3. The wound is closed in layers, and a posterior splint is applied with the ankle in neutral.

Postoperative Management. The splint is changed and the skin sutures removed at 10 to 14 days. A removable orthosis is applied, and motion exercises are allowed with protected weight-bearing after 4 weeks. After 6 weeks, shoewear can be resumed. Athletic activities are deferred until 8 weeks after surgery.

Excision of Lateral Talar Process Fracture

Technique

1. The procedure is the same as for open reduction and internal fixation, except: After exposing the fracture the fragment is sharply dissected from its ligamentous attachments. The ligaments are imbricated over the defect with 0 absorbable suture.

2. After closure a posterior splint is applied with the ankle in neutral.

Postoperative Management. The splint and sutures are removed at 10 to 14 days. An orthosis is applied, but motion exercises are not performed until 3 to 4 weeks after surgery. Protected weight-bearing is then allowed using the orthosis for an additional 3 weeks. Activities are advanced as tolerated.

Subtalar Dislocation

Most subtalar dislocations occur medially. They are the result of an inversion force, wherein the foot dislocates from the talus at

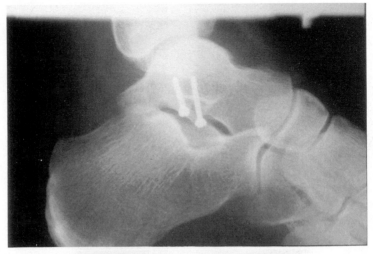

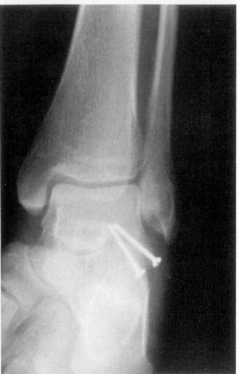

FIGURE 2.16. Internal fixation of the lateral process of a talus fracture.

the talocalcaneal and talonavicular articulations and is displaced medially. Lateral dislocations, resulting from an eversion force, are less common. Recognition of the characteristic foot deformity and an AP radiograph of the ankle confirm the diagnosis (Fig. 2.17). Lateral and oblique radiographs are helpful for excluding associated fractures. Skin tenting and neurovascular compromise can occur with this injury, making early reduction imperative. Late complications include recurrent instability, avascular necrosis of the talus, and degenerative arthritis of the subtalar joint.

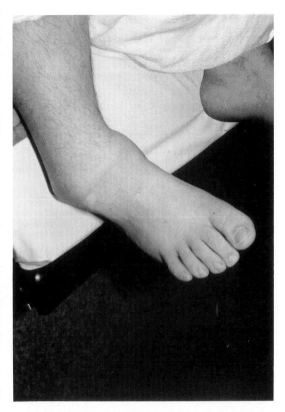

FIGURE 2.17. Clinical appearance of a medial subtalar dislocation.

Reduction

Closed reduction is usually possible by reversing the injury producing force. Apply gentle longitudinal traction to the forefoot with countertraction to the flexed knee and leg; exaggerate the deformity to unlock the dislocated bones and then apply either an eversion moment to the forefoot for medial dislocation or an inversion moment to the laterally dislocated foot. Reduction may be blocked by interlocked osteochondral fragments at the talonavicular joint or button-holing of the talus head through the extensor tendons (medial dislocation) or interposition of the posterior tibial tendon (lateral dislocation) (Buckingham, 1975; Leitner, 1954). If closed reduction is unsuccessful, a straight incision over the prominent talar neck and head, while protecting the dorsalis pedis and deep peroneal nerve laterally, allows extrication of the structures blocking reduction.

Postreduction Management

Use a short-leg cast and weight-bearing as tolerated to prevent redislocation and late instability. Casting should be continued for 3 weeks, followed by early motion exercises for the ankle and subtalar joints (DeLee and Curtis, 1982). Loss of subtalar motion is usual but is not typically limiting (Monson and Ryan, 1981). A program similar to that outlined for ankle fractures is utilized. Most patients can return to activities within 10 to 12 weeks of their injury.

Fracture of Dorsal Lip of the Navicular

Fracture of the dorsal lip of the navicular is an avulsion fracture that may be confused with an ankle sprain or a midfoot sprain (DeLee, 1993). It should be considered when evaluating presumed sprains that have not healed with conventional treatment. An accessory ossicle, the os talonavicularum, may be confused with an avulsion fracture.

Mechanism

The convex head of the talus articulates with the concave proximal navicular and is supported by ligaments dorsally and medially. The injury occurs with forced plantarflexion, usually combined with inversion. This mechanism may cause confusion with an inversion ankle sprain. The dorsal ligament is stronger than the bone that is avulsed.

Clinical Presentation

Point tenderness is maximal over the dorsal talonavicular joint, accompanied by swelling and ecchymosis. Careful examination of the ankle reveals minimal or no tenderness. Inversion of the ankle with the foot stabilized is well tolerated. Conversely, stabilizing the ankle and plantarflexing the midfoot elicits pain.

Radiography

The fracture can be discerned on a lateral view of the foot or ankle if it includes the talonavicular joint.

Treatment

This fracture can be treated satisfactorily with immobilization in a short-leg walking cast or walking orthosis for 3 to 4 weeks. Surgery can be considered if there is a residual symptomatic prominence over the joint.

References

Ahstrom JP: Spontaneous rupture of the plantar fascia. Am J Spaorts Med 16:306–307, 1988

Allenmark C: Partial achilles tendon tears. Clin Sports Med 11:759–769, 1992

Angermann P: Chronic retrocalcaneal bursitis treated by resection of the calcaneus. Foot Ankle 10:285–287, 1990

Anderson RB, Foster MD: Operative treatment of subcalcaneal pain. Foot Ankle 9:317–323, 1989

Barrett SL, Day SV: Endoscopic plantar fasciotomy for chronic plantar fasciitis/heel spur syndrome: surgical technique—early clinical results. J Foot Surg 30:568–570, 1991

Baxter DE, Thigpen CM: Heel pain—operative results. Foot Ankle 5:16–25, 1984

Berkowitz JF, Kier R, Rudicel S: Plantar fasciitis: MR imaging. Radiology 179:665–667, 1991

Bordelon RL: Heel pain. In: Mann RA, Coughlin MJ (eds): Surgery of the Foot and Ankle, Chapter 20, pp 837–847. St Louis, Mosby, 1993

Buckingham WW Jr: Subtalar dislocation of the foot. J Trauma 13:753–765, 1973

Cain MR, Baxter, DE: Achilles tendinitis. Foot Ankle 13:482–487,1992

Chandler TJ, Kibler WB: A biomechanical approach to the prevention, treatment and rehabilitation of plantar fasciitis. Sports Med 15:344–352, 1993

Clancy WG, Neidhart D, Brand RL: Achilles tendonitis in runners: a report of five cases. Am J Sports Med 4:46–56, 1976

Daly PJ, Kitaoka HB, Chao EYS: Plantar fasciotomy for intractable plantar fasciitis: clinical results and biomechanical evaluation. Foot Ankle 13:188–195, 1992

Davis PF, Severud E, Baxter DE: Painful heel syndrome: results of nonoperative treatment. Foot Ankle 15:531–535, 1994

DeLee, JC: Fractures and dislocations of the foot. In: Mann RA, Coughlin MJ (eds): Surgery of the Foot and Ankle, p 1465–1703. St. Louis, Mosby, 1993

DeLee JC, Curtis R: Subtalar dislocation of the foot. J Bone Joint Surg Am 64:433–437, 1982

Elkus RA: Tarsal coalition in the young athelete. Am J Sports Med 14:477–480, 1986

Fiamengo SA, Warren RF, Marshall JL, et al: Posterior heel pain associated with calcaneal step and achilles tendon calcification. Clin Orthop 167:203–211, 1982

Forman WM, Green MA: The role of intrinsic musculature in the formation of inferior calcausal exostoses. Clin Podiatr Med Surg 7:217–222, 1990

Fowler, A, Philip JF: Abnormality of the calcaneus as a cause of painful heel. Br J Surg 32:494–498, 1945

Frey C, Rosenberg Z, Shereff MJ, Kim H: The retrocalcaneal bursa: anatomy and bursography. Foot Ankle 13:203–207,1992

Gellman M: Fractures of the anterior process of the calcaneus. Bone Joint Surg Am 33:382–386, 1954

Gregg JR, Das M: Foot and ankle problems in the preadolescent and adolescent athlete. Clin Sports Med 1:131–147, 1982

Griffin LY: Common sports injuries of the foot and ankle seen in children and adolescents. Orthop Clin North Am 25:83–93, 1994

Hawkins LG: Fracture of the lateral process of the talus: a review of thirteen cases. J Bone Joint Surg Am 47:1170–1175, 1965

Heneghan MA, Pavlov H: The Haglund painful heel syndrome: experimental investigation of cause and therapeutic implications. Clin Orthop 187:228–234, 1984

Henricson AS, Westlin NE: Chronic calcaneal pain in athletes: entrapment of the calcaneal nerve? Am J Sports Med 12:152–154, 1984

Herrick RT, Herrick S: Rupture of the plantar fascia in a middle-aged tennis player: a case report. Am J Sports Med 11:95, 1983

Herzenberg JE, Goldner JL, Martinez S, Silverman PM: Computerized tomography of talocalcaneal tarsal coalition: a clinical and anatomic study. Foot Ankle 6:273–288, 1986

Hullinger CW: Insufficiency fracture of the calcaneus: similar to march fracture of the metatarsal. J Bone Joint Surg 26:751–757, 1944

Jahss MH, Kay BS: An anatomic study of the anterior superior process of the os calcis and its clinical application. Foot Ankle 3:269–281, 1983

Jahss MH, Michelson JD, Desai JD: Investigations into the fat pads of the sole of the foot: anatomy and histology. Foot Ankle 13:233–242, 1992

Kahn C, Bishop JO, Tullos HS: Plantar fascia release and heel spur excision via plantar route. Orthop Rev 14:222–225, 1985

Karr SD: Subcalcaneal heel pain. Orthop Clin North Am 25:161–175, 1994

Kitaoka HB, Luo ZP, Growney ES, et al: Material

properties of the plantar aponeurosis. Foot Ankle 15:557–560, 1994

Kwong PK, Kay D, Voner RT, White MW: Plantar fasciitis: mechanics and pathomechanics of treatment. Clin Sports Med 7:119–126, 1988

Leabhart JW: Stress fractures of the calcaneus. J Bone Joint Surg Am 41:1285–1290, 1959

Leach RE, DiIorio E, Harney RA: Pathologic hindfoot conditions in the athlete. Clin Orthop 177:116–121, 1983

Leach RE, Seavey MS, Salter DK: Results of surgery in athletes with plantar fasciitis. Foot Ankle 7:156–161, 1986

Leitner B: Obstacles to reduction in subtalar dislocations. J Bone Joint Surg Am 36:299–306, 1954

Lester DK, Buchanan JR: Surgical treatment of plantar fasciitis. Clin Orthop 186:202–204, 1984

Lewis G, Gatti A, Barry LD, et al: The plantar approach to heel surgery: a retrospective study. J Foot Surg 30:542–546, 1991

Lutter L: Surgical decisions in athletes' subcalcaneal pain. Am J Sports Med 14:481–485, 1986

McBryde AM: Plantar fasciitis. AAOS Instruct Course Lect 33:278–282, 1984

Micheli LJ, Ireland ML: Prevention and management of calcaneal apophysitis in children: an overuse syndrome. J Pediatr Orthop 7:34–38, 1987

Miller WE: The heel pad. Am J Sports Med 10:19–21, 1982

Monson ST, Ryan JR: Subtalar disloation. J Bone Joint Surg Am 63:1156–1158, 1981

Morgan RC, Crawford AH: Surgical management of tarsal coalition in adolescent athletes. Foot Ankle 7:183–193, 1986

Motto SG: Stress fracture of the lateral process of the talus—a case report. Br J Sports Med 27:275–276, 1993

Mukherjee SK, Pringle RM, Baxter AD: Fracture of the lateral process of the talus: a report of thirteen cases. J Bone Joint Surg Br 56:263–273, 1974

Nelen G, Martens, M, Burssens A: Surgical treatment of chronic achilles tendinitis. Am J Spaorts Med 17:754–759, 1989

O'Neill DB, Micheli LJ: Tarsal coalition: a followup of adolescent athletes. Am J Sports Med 17:544–549,1989

Pavlov H, Heneghan MA, Hersh A: The Haglund syndrome: initial and differential diagnosis. Diagn Radiol 144:83–88, 1982

Prichasuk S: The heel pad in plantar heel pain. J Bone Joint Surg Br 76:140–142, 1994

Rubin G, Witten M: Plantar calcaneal spurs. Am J Orthop 5:38, 1963

Sarrafian SK: Osteology: calcaneus. Antaomy of the Foot and Ankle, pp 54–62. Philadelphia, JB Lippincott CO, 1983

Schepsis AA, Leach RE, Gorzyca J: Plantar fasciitis: etiology, treatment, surgical results, and review of the literature. Clin Orthop 266:185–196, 1991

Schon LC, Glennon TP, Baxter DE: Heel pain syndrome: electrodiagnostic support for nerve entrapment. Foot Ankle 14:129–135, 1993

Scoli MW: Achilles tendinitis. Orthop Clin North Am 25:177–182, 1994

Sellman JR: Plantar fascia rupture associated with corticosteroid injection. Foot Ankle 15:376–381, 1994

Sewell JR, Black CM, Chapman AH, et al: Quantitative scintigraphy in diagnosis and management of plantar fasciitis (calcaneal periostitis): concise communication. J Nucl Med 21:663–666, 1980

Smart GW, Taunton JE, Clement DB: Achilles tendon disorders in runners—a review. Med Sci Sports Exerc 12:231–243,1980

Snider MP, Clancy WG, McBeath AA: Plantar fascia release for chronic plantar fasciitis in runners. Am J Sports Med 11:215–219, 1983

Snyder RB, Lipscomb AB, Johnston RK: The relationship of tarsal coalitions to ankle sprains in athletes. Am J Sports Med 9:313–317, 1981

Stephens MM: Haglund's deformity and retrocalcaneal bursitis. Orthop Clin North Am 25:41–45, 1994

Swiontkowski MF, Scranton PE, Hansen S: Tarsal coalitions: long-term results of surgical treatment. J Pediatr Orthop 3:287–292,1983

Tanz SS: Heel pain. Clin Orthop 28:169, 1963

Vasavada PJ, DeVries DF, Nishiyama H: Plantar fasciitis—early blood pool images in diagnosis of inflammatory process. Foot Ankle 5:74–76, 1984

Wall JR, Harkness MA, Crawford A: Ultrasound diagnosis of plantar fasciitis. Foot Ankle 14:465–470, 1993

Wapner KL, Sharkey PF: The use of night splints for treatment ofrecalcitrant plantar fasciitis. Foot Ankle 12:135–137, 1991

Warren BL: Plantar fasciitis in runners: treatment and prevention. Sports Med 10:338–345, 1990

Williams JGP: Achilles tendon lesions in sport. Sports Med 16:216–220, 1993

Williams PL, Smibert JG, Cox R, et al: Imaging study of the painful heel syndrome. Foot Ankle 7:345–349, 1987

Wolgin M, Cook C, Graham C, Mauldin D: Conservative treatment of plantar heel pain: long-term follow-up. Foot Ankle 15:97–102, 1994

3
Midfoot

Sprains

The spectrum of injury to the tarsometatarsal joints ranges from a mild sprain to frank dislocation. Dislocation of the tarsometatarsal joints is recognized as a significant injury, but lesser degrees of injury are often overlooked. Nonetheless, these "milder" injuries are often associated with prolonged symptoms and disability in the athlete.

Mechanism of Injury

Most of the athletic injuries of the tarsometatarsal joints are produced by indirect forces. Typically, a twisting force applied to the plantarflexed ankle and foot is responsible for injury (Meyer et al., 1994; Shapiro et al., 1994). An abduction force may be applied to the forefoot when the athlete pivots and the foot is fixed. A backward fall with the forefoot fixed, causing hyperplantarflexion of the forefoot has been described (Curtis et al., 1993). Less frequently, a direct blow to the dorsum of the midfoot is responsible.

Clinical Presentation

The athlete can usually describe the mechanism of the injury and reports generalized midfoot pain or pain localized medially, laterally, or centrally. With mild injury, weight-bearing may still be possible without pain.

Physical examination is most helpful for establishing the diagnosis (Curtis et al., 1993; Meyer et al.,1994; Shapiro et al., 1994). Swelling, although it may be subtle, and localized tenderness are the most frequent findings. Pain produced with medio-lateral compression, passive supination, and pronation of the midfoot are significant findings. Tenderness between the first and second metatarsals should be specifically sought on the examination. Functional tests including and inability to perform or the production of pain with single leg toe raise, jumping, and pivoting are suggestive of midfoot injury.

Radiography

Routine anteroposterior (AP) and lateral radiographs of the foot are usually negative. A weight-bearing AP view of the foot may, however, reveal widening of the first and second metatarsal interspace; and on occasion, an avulsion fracture is noted (Figs. 3.1, 3.2). A comparison view is usually necessary. A lateral radiograph is required to evaluate the longitudinal arch. Collapse is determined if the medial cuneiform is plantar to the base of the fifth metatarsal (Faciszewski et al., 1990). Especially with sprains that involve the medial tarsometatarsal joints, the lateral radiograph should be carefully reviewed to determine any collapse of the longitudinal arch (Fig. 3.3).

Treatment

Meyer et al. (1994) recognized the differences between isolated lateral tarsometatarsal

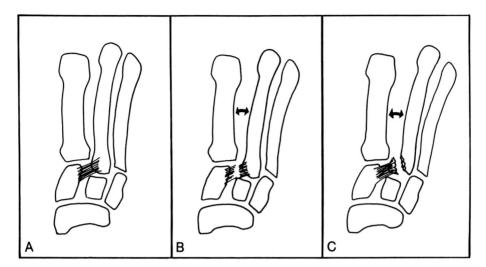

FIGURE 3.1. Injury to Lisfranc's ligament. (A) Lisfranc's ligament, attaching the base of the second metatarsal to the medial cuneiform. (B) Rupture of Lisfranc's ligament, causing diastasis between the first and second metatarsal bases. (C) Avulsion fracture occurs instead of ligament rupture.

sprains and those with medial involvement. Lateral sprains typically resolve quickly, whereas those with medial involvement are more severe and lead to prolonged disability. These authors recommended immobilization in a short-leg cast with protected ambulation as necessary for sprains involving the medial tarsometatarsal joints. Many lateral sprains were successfully treated by use of a rigid orthosis for the foot and ankle or a splint.

Typically, injuries with medial involvement require casting for up to 4 to 6 weeks. Regardless of the type or degree of injury, protection is necessary until repeat examination demonstrates an absence of tenderness. Return to activity follows a functional rehabilitation program to restore sport specific demands. A well molded arch support may be useful.

Radiographic changes dictate the need for treatment. Although slight widening of the first and second metatarsal interspace on the AP view has been reported to not cause long-term disability (Faciszewski et al., 1990), closed reduction (Fig. 3.4) and cast immobilization for a minimum of 4 weeks is safest, and operative reduction and fixation should be undertaken if uncertainty exists. If the lateral radiograph demonstrates collapse or sagging of the longitudinal arch, operative reduction and screw fixation to restore joint congruity is indicated to prevent a poor outcome.

Stress Fractures

Stress fractures account for nearly 5% of all sports injuries. Running is the sport most commonly involved, but these injuries also occur during basketball, dancing, and other sports that require repetitive jumping and sprinting. In the ankle and foot of athletes stress fractures of the fibula and distal tibia are most frequent, although clinically significant stress fractures occur also in the midfoot, affecting the tarsal navicular, proximal fifth metatarsal, and other metatarsal bases. Stress fractures that occur about the midfoot can be difficult to diagnose and treat, frequently requiring surgical intervention in the athlete.

Etiology

A number of factors have been implicated in the development of stress fractures including increases in frequency, duration, and intensity of activity—collectively referred to as "training errors." Additional associated fac-

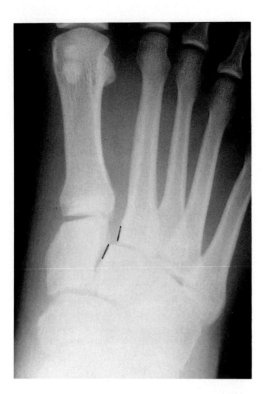

FIGURE 3.2. Midfoot sprain with injury to Lisfranc's ligament. Note the widening of the interval between the bases of the first and second metatarsals. The second metatarsal does not align with the middle cuneiform.

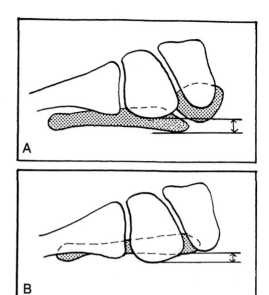

FIGURE 3.3. Flattening of the midfoot after a sprain. (A) Normal relation of the base of the medial cuneiform and the base of the fifth metatarsal. (B) Flattening of the midfoot causes the medial cuneiform to lie plantar to the fifth metatarsal. (After Faciszewski et al., 1990, with permission)

tors are alignment of the foot and type of shoewear. A positive correlation has been found between pronation of the foot and tarsal and tibial fractures as well as cavus foot deformity and metatarsal fractures.

Pathogenesis

Stress fractures are caused by the application of repetitive loads that exceed the ability of the bone to remodel. Lack or loss of muscle support, as occurs in the unconditioned or fatigued athlete, may be an important factor in the development of these injuries. The response to physical loads is both osteoclastic and osteoblastic. Li et al. (1985) have described the histologic changes in a unique experimental model. The initial event is vascular congestion accompanied by osteoclast-

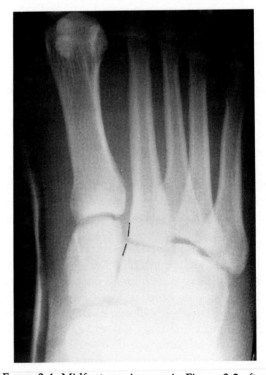

FIGURE 3.4. Midfoot sprain seen in Figure 3.2 after reduction by adduction and casting.

mediated bone resorption in the haversian canals and interstitial lamellae. Small cracks appear at the cement lines of the haversian canals and propagate into microfractures. Increased osteoblastic activity from the periosteum results in new bone formation. Stress fractures develop when osteoclastic activity exceeds the osteoblastic response.

Clinical Presentation

Infrequently symptoms develop after acute trauma. Most often pain occurs insidiously and increases gradually. At first, pain appears during activity and is relieved by rest. Subsequently, the pain intensifies, preventing activity, and may not be relieved by rest. A history of a recent increase in activity and training or a change in shoes and running surface may be noted.

Localized tenderness is characteristic; referred pain from distant percussion on the affected bone often can be elicited. Soft tissue swelling can be present, especially in the forefoot. Cavus deformity and pronation of the foot should be noted, as well as the range of motion of the ankle and subtalar joints.

Radiography

Diagnosis requires radiographic confirmation. For as long as 3 weeks after the onset of symptoms, however, routine radiographs may not demonstrate any abnormality, particularly for the tibia, fibula, calcaneus, and navicular. Usually, though, plain radiographs are sufficient to diagnose stress fractures of the metatarsals, including fracture of the proximal diaphysis of the fifth metatarsal. When routine radiographs are negative, technetium 99 scintigraphy is performed. Although not specific for the diagnosis, bone scanning is an extremely sensitive test for excluding a stress fracture (Prather et al., 1977). Focal activity on bone scan can be further studied with conventional tomography, computed tomography (CT), or magnetic resonance imaging (MRI) if anatomic visualization of the fracture is important (tarsal and metatarsal base fractures).

Treatment

Nonoperative and operative treatments are utilized depending on the area of involvement and the response to initial measures. In general, most stress fractures respond to avoidance of impact for 4 to 8 weeks combined with a program that allows maintenance of aerobic conditioning by bicycling, swimming, or water running. Resumption of impact activity is allowed in graduated fashion following the resolution of pain. This program effectively treats fractures of the distal tibia and fibula, calcaneus, and midshaft metatarsals.

Immobilization together with non-weight-bearing are necessary, at least, for stress fractures of the navicular and proximal diaphysis of the fifth metatarsal. Operative intervention is undertaken primarily for proximal diaphyseal fractures of the fifth metatarsal and for failure to heal with other fractures. Treatment of those stress fractures affecting the midfoot are discussed below. Stress fractures of the sesamoids are discussed in Chapter 2.

Fracture of the Proximal Diaphysis of the Fifth Metatarsal (Jones Fracture)

Jones fracture (Jones, 1902) may present as an acute traumatic event as evidenced by a pop and sharp pain, resulting in an inability to walk without a limp; or it may appear as a chronic condition associated with pain and impaired performance. Diagnosis is suggested by pain and tenderness localized over the plantar-lateral aspect of the proximal diaphysis of the fifth metatarsal.

Unlike other stress fractures, the Jones fracture is well demonstrated by routine radiographs (Fig. 3.5). In certain cases, intramedullary sclerosis and fracture widening are found, suggesting a remote or chronic condition that has progressed to nonunion (Fig. 3.6).

It is important to differentiate this fracture

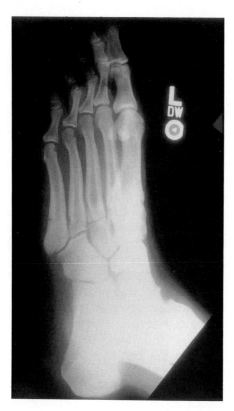

FIGURE 3.5. Acute Jones fracture of the fifth metatarsal.

weeks combined with strict non-weight-bearing can be successful. However, because of the high success rate and minimal morbidity of intramedullary screw fixation, it is our preferred approach for managing the acute fracture (Mindrebo et al., 1993). On rare occasions the fracture is found to be nonunited, and curettage and bone grafting are necessary (Torg, et al., 1984), which can be combined with intramedullary screw fixation if desired.

Intramedullary Screw Fixation

Technique

1. General, epidural, or regional block anesthesia can be used. The patient is positioned supine on a radiolucent table top with a bump placed underneath the ipsilateral hip to internally rotate the lower

from avulsion of the tuberosity of the fifth metatarsal by the action of the peroneus brevis, which results from an inversion injury to the ankle and foot (Fig. 3.7). Avulsion injuries usually heal rapidly with taping or casting and without residual sequelae. Delayed and non-union of Jones fractures can occur, with vascular insufficiency (Smith, 1991) an important factor.

Treatment

Four therapeutic options exist: benign neglect, plaster immobilization with or without electrical stimulation (Holmes, 1884) intramedullary lag screw fixation, and inlay bone grafting. If the injury is chronic and symptoms are minimal, the athlete may elect to continue to play for the remainder of the season, at which time surgery can be performed. In the recreational athlete with an acute injury, plaster immobilization for 6 to 8

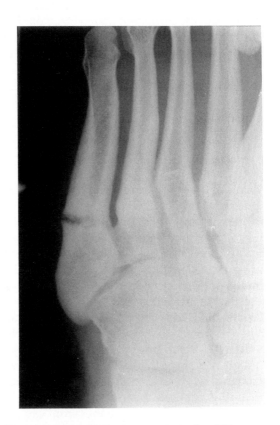

FIGURE 3.6. Established nonunion of a fifth metatarsal Jones fracture. Note fracture widening and intramedullary sclerosis.

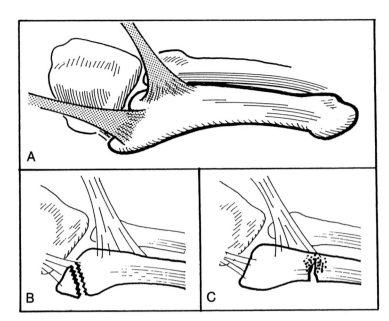

FIGURE 3.7. Patterns of proximal fifth metatarsal fractures. (A) Peroneus brevis and peroneus tertius attachments to the base of the fifth metatarsal. (B) Avulsion fracture (dancer's fracture). (C) Jones fracture.

extremity, facilitating access to the lateral border of the foot.

2. Under tourniquet control a 3 cm straight incision is made in line with the longitudinal axis of the fifth metatarsal, starting at the base of the tuberosity and extending proximally.

3. Incise the subcutaneous tissue, protecting any branches of the sural nerve. Dorsally, identify the peroneus tertius and brevis tendons as they insert on the base of the fifth metatarsal.

4. Using image intensification, insert a 3.2 mm drill bit starting at the tip of the tuberosity in line with the longitudinal axis of the metatarsal. Adduction of the forefoot is helpful for exposing the base of the metatarsal. A cannulated system, which allows placement of an initial guidewire, can be used as well.

5. Drill past the fracture to the proposed length of the screw. Make sure that the threads of the selected 4.5 mm malleolar screw engage only in the canal distal to the fracture (Fig. 3.8).

6. Do not countersink the screw head in order to achieve maximum compression.

7. If the canal is large and firm purchase is not obtained with the 4.5 mm screw, redrill the canal with a 4.5 mm drill bit and

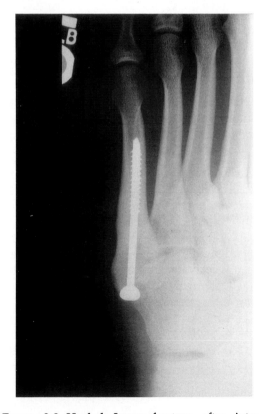

FIGURE 3.8. Healed Jones fracture after intramedullary fixation with a 4.5 mm AO malleolar screw.

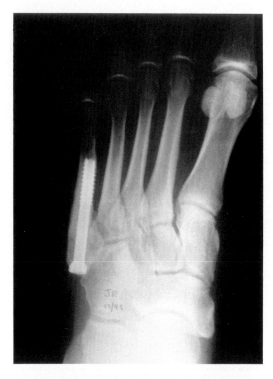

FIGURE 3.9. Fixation with a 6.5 mm lag screw.

control, make a 5 cm straight incision along the lateral border of the fifth metatarsal, centered over the tuberosity.

2. Protect any sensory branches from the sural nerve while developing the deeper dissection along the inferior border of the peroneus brevis tendon. Expose the fracture site by incising the periosteum.

3. Trim sclerotic ends of the fracture with a small rongeur and curet. Outline a rectangular trough centered over the fracture, perforating the lateral cortex cortex, and remove this block (Figs. 3.10A,B).

4. Using a template of the trough or the removed bone itself, harvest a corresponding piece of corticocancellous bone graft from the iliac crest or distal medial tibia, which is 2 mm larger in all directions. Additional cancellous graft is also harvested.

insert the appropriate length 6.5 mm cancellous screw (Fig. 3.9).

8. Close only the skin with interrupted mattress sutures using 3–0 nylon and apply a well padded posterior or U-splint to the foot, ankle, and leg.

Postoperative Management. No weight-bearing is allowed until approximately 2 weeks, at which time the splint and sutures are removed and the patient is fitted with a CAM walker. Progressive increase in weight-bearing is allowed over the next 3 to 4 weeks. At 6 weeks resistive exercises for the ankle and foot can be started, and the patient is allowed to ambulate in an athletic shoe.

Healing is usually apparent radiographicaly by 8 weeks, and return to activity occurs by 8 to 12 weeks. Orthotics are not necessary unless significant foot deformity is present.

Bone Grafting Alone or With Internal Fixation

Technique

1. Using an anesthetic and positioning as described above and under tourniquet

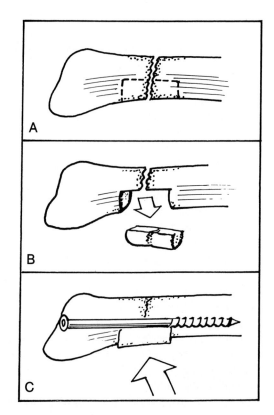

FIGURE 3.10. Bone grafting of a Jones fracture. (A) Jones fracture with the segment to be excised outlined. (B) Excision of a rectangular segment containing the fracture. (C) Bone graft is in place with supplemental screw fixation.

5. The cancellous graft is placed in the fracture site, and the corticocancellous block that has been fashioned is press-fit into the trough spanning the fracture (Fig. 3.11).

6. At this point, the wound can be closed; or, if desired, supplemental intramedullary screw fixation can be performed to achieve a "belt and suspenders" construct (Fig. 3.10C). In either instance, close the wound as described above.

Postoperative Management. Because this procedure is used more often for established non-unions, healing is slower than for acute fractures without sclerosis. Protected weight-bearing and immobilization are used for 6 to 8 weeks. Return to sports activity usually requires 12 to 14 weeks.

Open Reduction of Intraarticular Fifth Metatarsal Base Fracture (Dancer's Fracture)

On occasion, an avulsion fracture of the fifth metatarsal tuberosity remains symptomatic despite nonoperative treatment. In such cases, fixation or excision is necessary.

Technique

1. With anesthesia and positioning similar to that described above, a 3 cm incision is made along the superior edge of the peroneus brevis tendon, centered over the dorsal aspect of the tuberosity. The sural nerve must be identified and protected.

2. The cuboid-metatarsal joint is entered dorsally and the fracture inspected. After irrigation to remove fracture fragments from the joint, the fracture is reduced, restoring joint congruity. Temporary fixation is performed with one or more 0.062 inch K-wires.

3. In most instances fixation is achieved with a small fragment cancellous screw. If not, the K-wires are left in place, and the wound is closed with the K-wires protruding through the skin.

4. The wound is closed in layers, and a posterior splint is applied.

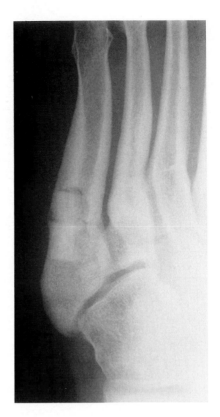

FIGURE 3.11. Radiograph after excision of a fracture and replacement with a corticocancellous bone block.

Postoperative Management

Protected weight-bearing with crutches is used for 10 to 14 days. Sutures are removed at that time. If screw fixation was used, weight-bearing is allowed with a removable walking orthosis for 4 weeks. If a K-wire was used, non-weight-bearing should continue for four additional weeks until the wire is removed in an outpatient setting. In both instances, shoewear and activities are begun 6 weeks after surgery if there is radiographic evidence of bone healing. Athletic activities can be resumed as rapidly as the ankle and foot regain full strength and motion.

Atypical Metatarsal Stress Fractures

Rarely, metatarsal stress fractures do not heal completely (Fig 3.12). Moreover, refracture may occur when the player returns to sport. In such instances, operative treatment is in-

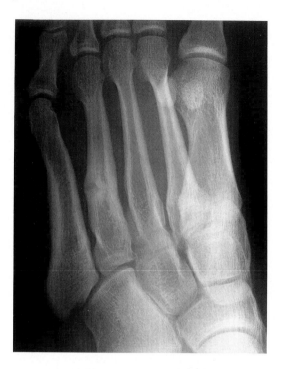

FIGURE 3.12. Painful metatarsal stress fracture incompletely healed. Note the cystic formation despite cast immobilization.

dicated. We prefer to manage this problem with bone grafting, plating, and interfragmentary screw fixation when possible. Union is usually complete by 10 to 12 weeks, and the athlete can return to activity by 4 months.

Stress fractures of the base of the metatarsals are infrequent but pose diagnostic and therapeutic challenges. Vague midfoot pain and normal routine radiographs are typical. Bone scans and MRI or CT are necessary to establish the diagnosis (Figs. 3.13, 3.14). Despite cast immobilization, union may not occur.

Nonetheless, we have long term follow-up on two patients who have remained symptom-free despite only fibrous union while continuing football and basketball, respectively. A well molded, semirigid orthosis has been helpful in both. For persistent symptoms, however, bone grafting is indicated.

Tarsal Navicular Stress Fracture

Tarsal navicular stress fractures have been reported to be among the most difficult to

diagnose and treat successfully (Torg et al., 1982). A history of trauma and other factors, including excessive pronation of the foot, limited ankle dorsiflexion, limited subtalar motion, shortening of the first metatarsal, or lengthened second metatarsal, combined with relative hypovascularity of the central portion of the navicular have been implicated in the development of tarsal navicular stress fractures.

Clinical Presentation

Symptoms are frequently insidious and vague, and radiographs are normal. Diagnosis requires a technetium 99 bone scan and conventional tomography to delineate the fracture (Figs. 3.15, 3.16). Acute, nondisplaced fractures are initially treated by non-weight-bearing and cast immobilization for 8 weeks. Surgical treatment is necessary for fractures that are displaced or fail to heal with immobilization. Although excision and en

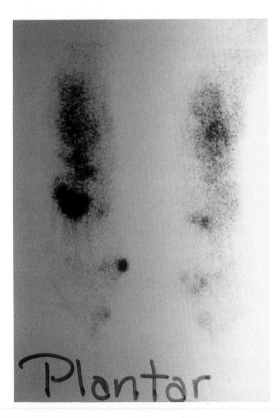

FIGURE 3.13. Intense uptake on a bone scan over the proximal middle metatarsals.

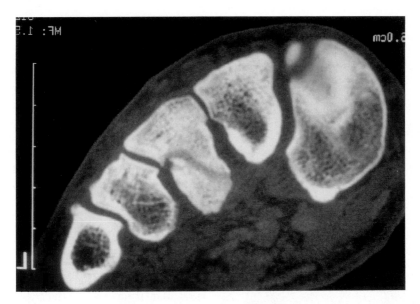

FIGURE 3.14. CT scan confirming a stress fracture in the base of the third metatarsal.

bloc bone grafting has been used for this injury (Fitch et al., 1989), compression with screw fixation is reliable and allows earlier return to activity.

ORIF of Tarsal Navicular Stress Fracture

Technique

1. Position the patient supine, using a radiolucent table for intraoperative radiography or image intensification. Utilize a tourniquet for improved visualization.

2. Make a dorsal, longitudinal incision over the middle third of the navicular, centered between the interval of the tibialis anterior and extensor hallucis longus tendons. Identify and retract laterally the deep peroneal nerve and dorsalis pedis artery.

3. By palpation and image intensification, identify the fracture site, elevating the periosteum to allow approximation of the fracture edges.

4. Ideally, insert two parallel 2 mm guidewires from a medial or lateral approach

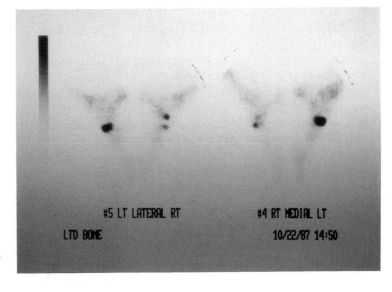

FIGURE 3.15. Focal uptake on a bone scan over the navicular.

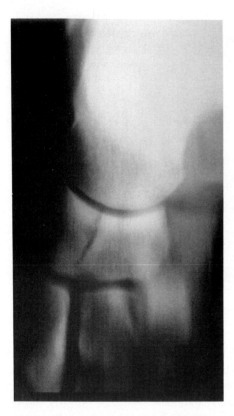

FIGURE 3.16. Tomogram demonstrating a navicular fracture.

and insert appropriate length 4.0 mm cannulated lag screws, ensuring that no screw threads cross the fracture. Sometimes only one screw can be inserted. It is occasionally necessary, especially when the fracture involves the extreme lateral one-third of the navicular, to cut off distal screw threads or consider fixation across the navicular into the cuboid to prevent having screw threads crossing the fracture.
5. Cancellous grafting from the iliac crest is used if the fracture edges are not compressed, but it is usually not necessary.
6. The skin is closed with interrupted simple mattress sutures (3–0 nylon), and a well padded posterior or U-splint is applied.

Postoperative Management

Remove the sutures at 10 to 14 days and replace the splint with a short-leg cast. Non-weight-bearing is instituted for 4 weeks, fol-lowed by protected weight-bearing in a cast or CAM walker for another 4 weeks. At 8 weeks, once the area is no longer tender and the patient walks without a limp, resistive exercises are started for the foot and ankle. Bicycling is helpful for regaining range of motion. Running is not permitted until there is radiographic evidence of healing. Tomography may be necessary to demonstrate bony healing. Return to sports requires a minimum of 3 months (usually 4–6 months).

Accessory Navicular

The accessory navicular is a supernumerary bone associated with the medial pole of the navicular. It has also been called the os tibiale externum, prehallux, and accessory scaphoid. The condition is found in 4% to 14% of the population and may occur unilaterally or bilaterally (Grogan et al., 1989). In most cases they are asymptomatic, but symptoms can arise owing to disruption of a synchondrosis with the navicular or irritation against the side of the shoe. The accessory navicular is contained in the insertional fibers of the posterior tibialis tendon, resulting in both tensile and compression forces being exerted on the accessory bone (Sella and Lawson, 1987).

Clinical Presentation

Children and adults with all three types of accessory navicular may have symptoms, depending on the size of the prominence (Fig. 3.17). The symptoms are usually due to rubbing against the side of the shoe but may be secondary to the prominence being kicked or otherwise acutely traumatized.

A second cause of symptoms is disruption of the fibers that attach the unfused accessory bone to the body of the navicular. This problem occurs in children and adults, usually following an acute twisting injury in which the accessory navicular is wrenched away from the navicular. Alternatively, the pain appears insidiously as a result of chronic irritation of the synchondrosis. Pain may radiate proximally along the course of the posterior tibialis tendon.

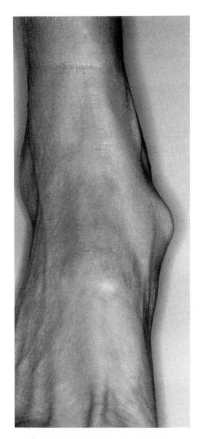

FIGURE 3.17. Accessory navicular. Note the prominence over the medial pole of the navicular due to an accessory navicular.

Radiography

Routine radiographs of the foot reveal an accessory navicular (Fig. 3.18). An external oblique view demonstrates the profile of the medial aspect of the navicular and is helpful for assessing the characteristics of an accessory navicular (Grogan et al., 1989).

The accessory navicular arises from a secondary center of ossification of the navicular medial to the usual one. In children the two centers have the radiographic appearance of being separate bones. Three patterns of accessory navicular are seen in adults (Fig. 3.19): Type I is a true sesamoid lying within the substance of the posterior tibialis tendon. A type II accessory bone has a cartilaginous synchondrosis with the medial navicular that is 1 to 3 mm in thickness. Type III is united to the medial pole of the navicular with a bridge

of bone (Sella and Lawson, 1987; Sella et al., 1986). Of the accessory naviculars, 30% are type I and 70% are type II or III (Sella and Lawson, 1987). Bone scanssare helpful for identifying a traumatized type II accessory navicular if plain radiographs are equivocal.

Nonoperative Treatment

When symptoms are related to friction of the prominence against the shoe, treatment is directed at pressure relief. Pads may be helpful, as may stretching the portion of the shoe overlying the prominence. If this treatment is unsatisfactory, surgical excision can be considered.

The initial treatment for pain from a synchondrosis is similar to that for a sprain. It includes rest and nonsteroidal antiinflammatory drugs (NSAIDs). Other modalities include a period of non-weight-bearing with crutches or immobilization in a short-leg walking cast for 3 to 6 weeks. Persistent symptoms warrant surgical treatment.

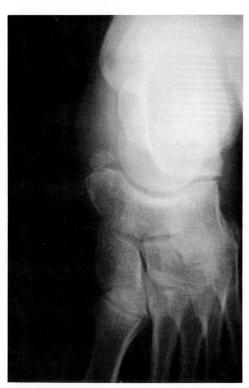

FIGURE 3.18. Type II accessory navicular with displacement.

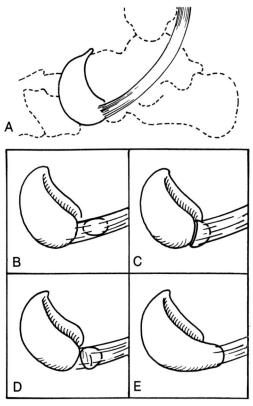

FIGURE 3.19. Accessory navicular. (A) Posterior tibial tendon inserts on navicular. (B) Type I. (C) Type II. (D) Type II, with displacement. (E) Type III.

Operative Treatment

The surgical procedure is the same for all types, regardless of the cause of symptoms. It consists in removing of the accessory navicular bone and the medial pole of the navicular and imbricating of the posterior tibialis tendon without rerouting the tendon. This procedure has produced excellent results in children and adults with an expectation of complete return to athletic activities (Grogan et al., 1989; Lepore et al., 1990; Sella and Lawson, 1987; Sella et al., 1986).

Excision of Accessory Navicular

Technique

1. A general anesthetic is administered and a thigh tourniquet applied. The skin incision follows the distal course of the posterior tibialis tendon from the inferior border of the medial malleolus to the medial pole of the navicular, extending to the level of the medial cuneiform.
2. The sheath of the posterior tibialis is entered proximally and split longitudinally until the insertion is well visualized over the entire medial pole.
3. A no. 15 scalpel is used to make a longitudinal cut in the distal 2 to 3 cm of the tendon, extending to the bone of the accessory navicular and the navicular proper.
4. The accessory bone is subperiosteally excised from the tendon, being careful not to transect fibers of the tendon. Dorsal and plantar elevation of the tendon insertion into the navicular is required to expose the medial pole. A small osteotome can then divide it parallel to the medial side of the foot. The edges are smothed with a rongeur and rasp.
5. The split in the tendon is repaired with a running stitch of 2–0 absorbable suture, starting proximally and continuing over the medial side of the navicular. The tendon sheath is closed with a running stitch of 0 absorbable suture.
6. The skin is closed with interrrupted 3–0 nylon mattress sutures, and a short-leg posterior or U-shaped splint is applied.

Postoperative Management

Protected weight-bearing is used for 10 to 14 days. The splint and skin sutures are removed, and a short-leg walking cast is applied for 4 weeks. After the cast is removed, walking is allowed in a regular shoe. Activities are advanced after 2 weeks, and training can resume 2 weeks later.

Plantar Fibromatosis

Plantar fibromatosis is a benign but locally aggressive tumor that forms in the plantar fascia. Microscopic examination of nodules shows a similarity with the tissue found in Dupuytren's contracture, the characteristic cell being a myofibroblast. The nodule appears without preceding trauma and is usually painless when small. After a variable time the nodule may begin to grow, at which point it may become painful and make shoewear and activities difficult. It can become locally aggressive and extend into the overlying fat and skin or the underlying muscle (Haedicke and Sturim, 1989).

Clinical Presentation

Plantar fibromatosis typically appears as a solitary nodule in the arch that is seen just underneath the skin. It may be tender to palpation, though these nodules are often asymptomatic. With more advanced cases multiple nodules can occur. Radiographs and MRI are not helpful for the diagnosis.

Treatment

Surgery is indicated when the nodule is painful or demonstrates significant growth. These lesions have a tendency to recur, so the excision must be extralesional. Because the skin flaps elevated in the area of resection are thin, care must be taken during the procedure to handle them carefully. Non-weight-bearing should be maintained for 3 weeks after surgery to ensure that the wound heals without shear forces on the edges.

Surgical Excision

1. The procedure is usually performed with the patient in the prone position, which requires a general anesthetic with intubation or an ankle block. A thigh tourniquet is used with a general anesthetic, and a Esmarch bandage at the ankle is used as a tourniquet with an ankle block.
2. The skin incision is centered over the nodule, running longitudinally on the plantar surface of the foot. It should extend 2 to 3 cm on either side of the nodule. The skin is thin under the arch, and there is little subcutaneous fat. The incision is carried down to the plantar fascia before any flaps are elevated, thereby ensuring that the entire thickness of the subcutaneous layer is included in the flap. The nodule is thus exposed.
3. A no. 15 scalpel is used to divide the fascia around the nodule with approximately a 1 cm rim of normal appearing fascia included in the specimen. The specimen is then elevated from the underlying muscle tissue (Fig. 3.20). Histologic examination is recommended.
4. The tourniquet is removed and hemostasis obtained with electrocautery. The incision is closed in layers with absorbable 3-0 approximating the subcutaneous layer, and the skin is closed with simple stitches of 3-0

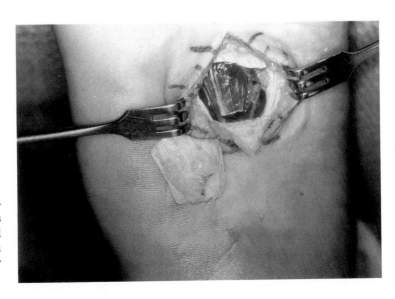

FIGURE 3.20. Plantar fibromatosis. A plantar fibroma was excised through a longitudinal incision. The fibroma with a margin of normal plantar fascia is shown.

nonabsorbable suture. A soft dressing is applied.

Postoperative Management

The patient is instructed to remain non-weight-bearing, using crutches for 3 weeks. The dressing is removed at 1 week, and bathing is allowed. Sutures are removed at 2 weeks. Initial weight-bearing is restricted to walking only for 7 to 10 days; activities are then advanced as tolerated.

References

Curtis MJ, Myerson M, Szuba, B: Tarsometatarsal joint injuries in the athlete. Am J Sports Med 21:497–502, 1993

Faciszewski T, Burks RT, Manaster BJ: Subtle injuries of the Lisfranc joint. J Bone Joint Surg Am 72:1519–1522, 1990

Fitch KD, Blackwell JB, Gilmour WN: Operation for nonunion of stress fractures of the tarsal navicular. J Bone Joint Surg Br 71:105–110, 1989

Grogan DP, Gasser SI, Ogden JA: The painful accessory navicular: a clinical and histopathological study. Food Ankle 10:164–169, 1989

Haedicke GJ, Sturim HS: Plantar fibromatosis: an isolated disease. Plast Reconstruct Surg 83:296–299, 1989

Holmes GB: Treatment of delayed unions and nonunions of the proximal fifth metatarsal with pulsed electromagnetic fields. Foot Ankle 15:552–556, 1884

Jones R: Fracture of the base of the fifth metatarsal by indirect violence. Ann Surg 35:697–702, 1902

Lepore L, Francobandiera C, Maffulli N: Fracture of the os tibiale externum in a decathlete. J Foot Surg 29:366–368, 1990

Li G, Zhang S, Chen G, et al: Radiographic and histologic analysis of stress fractures in rabbit tibias. Am J Sports Med 13:285, 1985

Meyer SA, Callaghan JJ, Albright JP, et al: Midfoot sprains in collegiate football players. Am J Sports Med 22:392–401, 1994

Mindrebo N, Shelbourne D, Van Meter CD, Retig AC: Outpatient percutaneous screw fixation of the acute Jones fracture. Am J Sports Med 21:720–723, 1993

Prather JL, Jusynowitz ML, Snowdy HA, et al: Scintigraphic findings in stress fractures. J Bone Joint Surg Am 59:869–874, 1977

Sella EJ, Lawson JP: Biomechanics of the accessory navicular synchondrosis. Foot Ankle 8:156–163, 1987

Sella EJ, Lawson JP, Ogden JA: The accessory navicular synchondrosis. Clin Orthop 209:280–285, 1986

Shapiro MS, Wascher DC, Finerman GAM: Rupture of Lisfranc's ligament in Athletes. Am J Sports Med 22:687–691, 1994

Smith JW, Arnoczky SP, Hersh A: The intraosseous blood supply of the fifth metatarsal: implications for proximal fracture healing. Foot Ankle 13:143–152, 1992

Torg JS, Balduini FC, Zelko RR, et al: Fractures of the base of the fifth metatarsal distal to the tuberosity. J Bone Joint Surg Am 66:209–214, 1984

Torg JS, Pavlov H, Cooley LH: Stress fractures of the tarsal navicular: a retrospective review of twenty-one cases. J Bone Joint Surg Am 63:700, 1982

4
Forefoot

Great Toe

The great toe and its metatarsophalangeal (MTP) joint are affected by numerous injuries, that in turn affect athletic performance. During the last phase of stance in the gait cycle, the body's weight is transferred forward onto the ball of the foot and the toes. From heel rise to toe-off during barefoot gait, the first MTP joint dorsiflexes with the joint subjected to a force 0.8 times body weight (McBride et al., 1991). Progressively decreasing forces are measured at the second through fifth MTP joints. First MTP joint forces are increased severalfold during athletic activities that involve running and jumping. The crouched position of a baseball catcher and the en pointe position of a ballet dancer are examples of high stress that occurs at the first MTP joint during athletics (Teitz et al., 1985). Such stress can lead to both acute and chronic injuries of the great toe.

Anatomy and Function

The hallux is extended by the action of the extensor hallucis longus, whose tendon attaches at the dorsal base of the distal phalanx. Flexion is accomplished by the flexor hallucis longus, inserting on the plantar aspect of the distal phalanx, and the flexor hallucis brevis, which inserts by two tendons on the plantar base of the proximal phalanx.

There are three sesamoid bones associated with the great toe, two of which are invariably present under the first metatarsal head and a third, which occurs in approximately 15% of the population, on the plantar aspect of the interphalangeal joint (Sarrafian, 1983). The interphalangeal sesamoid lies in the flexor hallucis longus tendon and is clinically insignificant. The MTP joint sesamoids articulate with the metatarsal by a distinct groove, and these grooves are separated by a midline prominence, the crista, on the plantar surface of the metatarsal head.

The MTP joint sesamoids are each embedded in the thick plantar plate of the first MTP joint. This structure is contiguous with the medial and lateral sesamophalangeal and metatarsosesamoid ligaments and an intersesamoid ligament. This complex of ligaments maintains the sesamoids and proximal phalanx in apposition to the metatarsal head during joint motion.

The tendons of the flexor hallucis contain the vascular supply to the sesamoids (Sobel et al., 1992). The lateral sesamoid receives insertions from the deep transverse metatarsal ligament and the oblique and transverse heads of the adductor hallucis. The abductor hallucis attaches to the medial sesamoid. The fibrous tunnel of the flexor hallucis longus tendon, which runs between the sesamoids, has attachments to both, as does the plantar fascia.

The medial sesamoid may be bipartite or multipartite (Richardson, 1987). Partite sesamoids are present in 10% to 30% of the population (Sarrafian, 1983; Scranton, 1981; Scranton and Rutkowski, 1980). They can occur unilaterally or bilaterally.

The sesamoids have an important role in the function of the first MTP joint. Foremost, they absorb impact, dispersing forces during weight-bearing, thereby protecting the first metatarsal head and the tendon of the flexor hallucis longus. They also function as a fulcrum to increase the moment arm of the flexor hallucis brevis muscle, increasing the power of first MTP plantarflexion.

Injuries of the Sesamoids

With their vulnerable position and the high stress to which the sesamoids are subjected, it is remarkable that injuries are not more common. When they do occur, however, these injuries can be disabling for the athlete. Such types of sesamoid injuries include sesamoiditis, stress fractures, and acute fractures.

Sesamoiditis

Sesamoiditis, or inflammation of the sesamoid complex, includes synovitis, flexor hallucis longus tendonitis, and chondromalacia of the sesamoid (Leventen, 1991; McBryde and Anderson, 1988). It usually develops insidiously as the result of chronic loading activities (Axe and Ray, 1988). Direct impact or the tensile forces generated during dorsiflexion of the MTP joint can initiate inflammation, and repeated minor trauma eventually causes symptoms (Dietzen, 1990).

Clinical Presentation

The athlete complains of pain upon weight-bearing along the ball of the foot, which can severely limit activities. It is unusual for the pain to occur along the medial eminence, as is noted with a bunion. Typically, the history is of a gradual onset of pain with no particular identifiable precipitating episode.

Physical examination reveals tenderness to palpation under the sesamoids, with one sometimes be more severely affected. Slight swelling may be seen on the plantar surface of the joint, but there is no ecchymosis or erythema. Passive range of motion can be

limited and painful, particularly in dorsiflexion. Axial compression of the surfaces of the MTP joint does not cause pain.

Radiography

Routine anteroposterior (AP) and lateral radiographs of the foot are usually normal, as are axial views of the sesamoids (Fig. 4.1). A technetium 99 bone scan may show tracer uptake in the area of the first MTP (Axe and Ray, 1988; Richardson, 1987).

Treatment

The primary mode of treatment is rest, which relieves inflammation. Limiting first MTP joint motion diminishes tensile forces in the sesamoid complex and can be accomplished by wearing shoes with a stiffened forefoot.

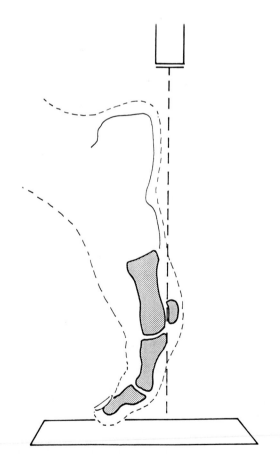

FIGURE 4.1. Correct position of the foot for obtaining a sesamoid radiograph. (After Richardson, 1987, with permission)

Taping of the great toe can also restrict dorsiflexion and may provide enough support to allow athletic activities to be continued. A felt HAPAD or metatarsal bar placed proximal to the MTP transfers weight-bearing pressure from the joint, reducing impact stress. Oral nonsteroidal antiinflammatory medications (NSAIDs) are helpful in patients who can tolerate them. Return to athletics is determined by the level of pain.

If pain continues, enforced rest of the foot is obtained by use of a short-leg walking cast for 2 to 4 weeks. The cast should have an extended toe plate to prevent motion at the MTP joint and a walking heel under the arch, which transfers weight-bearing forces from the ball of the foot.

A single intraarticular injection of cortisone can provide substantial or complete relief of symptoms in the recalcitrant case. The injection is performed with cast immobilization for 2 to 4 weeks.

Custom orthotic treatment permits early return to sport participation (Axe and Ray, 1988). The device should be full length to prevent overpronation, with a J-shaped pad incorporated to provide sesamoid stress relief.

If these treatment modalities do not relieve pain over 4 to 6 months, sesamoidectomy is considered (Richardson, 1987).

Acute Sesamoid Fracture

Acute sesamoid fractures can occur by two mechanisms. A direct blow to the medial ball of the foot can compress the sesamoid against the metatarsal head, which occurs during a fall from some height or from a hard landing on the ball of the foot with compression of the sesamoid. Runners, dancers, and basketball players may sustain the injury in this manner. The sesamoid may also fracture under tension. When the great toe is violently dorsiflexed, the sesamoid is pulled apart (McBryde and Anderson, 1988). The medial sesamoid is most commonly involved, probably because of its shape and the fact that the lateral sesamoid is often partly displaced lateral to the metatarsal head (Irvin et al., 1985).

Clinical Presentation

Because an acute sesamoid fracture follows an identifiable traumatic event the athlete should be able to describe the mechanism of injury. Clinically, there is swelling and often ecchymosis on the plantar aspect of the first MTP joint. The area is tender to palpation, and dorsiflexion of the MTP is painful.

Radiography

Appropriate radiographs include AP, oblique, and lateral views of the foot and an axial view of the sesamoids. The diagnosis can usually be confirmed by these studies (Fig. 4.1). The main distinctions that must be made are between an acute fracture, a partite sesamoid, and osteonecrosis of the sesamoid (Fig. 4.2).

An acute fracture demonstrates irregular edges, whereas a partite sesamoid has smooth, regular edges that are usually sclerotic. An osteonecrotic sesamoid is fragmented into multiple pieces, and there may

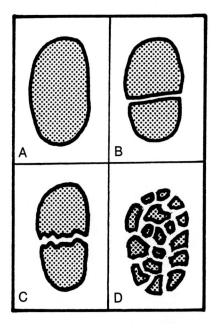

FIGURE 4.2. Variations in the sesamoids. (A) Normal appearance. (B) Bipartite sesamoid with smooth borders. (C) Sesamoid fracture with irregular borders. (D) Fragmented sesamoid, osteochondritis.

be remodeling of the sesamoid and the metatarsal head with new bone formation. The
axial radiograph may demonstrate fracture of
the sesamoid (Fig. 4.3). If not, a technetium
99 bone scan is performed to identify the
acute fracture.

Nonoperative Treatment

Sesamoid fractures may require a prolonged
time to heal, and the athlete should be in-
formed of this problem at the beginning of
treatment. If symptoms are mild, treatment
employs the modalities used for sesamoiditis:
taping, metatarsal pads, and a stiff-soled
shoe. If significant pain is present, a short-leg
walking cast is used for 4 to 6 weeks. The cast
should have an extended toe plate to prevent
MTP joint motion and a posteriorly placed
heel pad to transfer weight-bearing from the
ball of the foot. The athlete is then advanced
to a stiff-soled shoe with a metatarsal pad to
relieve the sesamoid (Fig. 4.4). The latter
device may be necessary for up to 4 to 6
months.

Operative Treatment

Significantly displaced sesamoid fractures
and nondisplaced fractures that do not respond to nonoperative treatment of 6 to 8
weeks can be considered for excision. The
medial sesamoid is excised through a medial
incision, and the lateral sesamoid is approached through a plantar incision (Leventen, 1991).

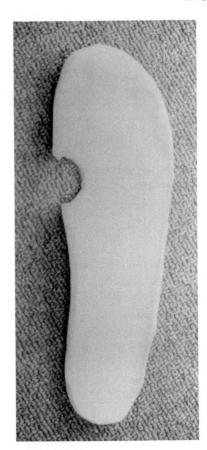

FIGURE 4.4. Sesamoid cut-out insole to relieve a
painful medial sesamoid.

Medial Sesamoidectomy

Technique

1. General anesthesia or an ankle block is
   used. Under tourniquet control, a 4 cm
   longitudinal incision is made on the infe-
   romedial aspect of the first ray, centered
   on the MTP joint. Care must be taken to
   prevent injury to the medial plantar sensory nerve to the hallux.
2. The MTP joint capsule is entered longitudinally in its plantar one-third, and the
   sesamoid and MTP joint surfaces are inspected. A no.15 scalpel is used to excise
   the medial sesamoid subperiosteally (Fig.
   4.5). The sesamoid is larger than it appears
   on the radiographs. If the flexor hallucis
   brevis tendon is damaged during the excision, it should be repaired with a 2–0
   absorbable suture, as should any defect in
   the plantar capsule.

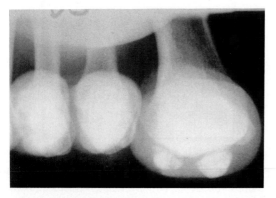

FIGURE 4.3. Fracture of the fibular sesamoid. Irregularities are seen in the lateral sesamoid.

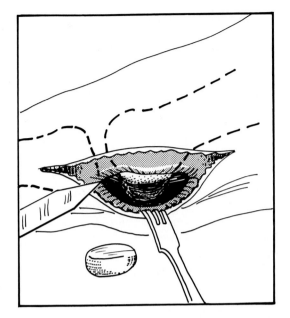

FIGURE 4.5. Excision of the medial sesamoid. The sesamoid is excised from its soft tissue attachments through a midline approach.

3. The wound is closed in layers to ensure that there is no medial laxity that could lead to the development of hallux valgus. A soft dressing is applied.

Postoperative Management. Immediate weight-bearing is allowed as tolerated with a postoperative shoe and crutches. The dressings are changed and sutures removed at 10 to 14 days. Walking is then allowed in a regular shoe, but athletic activities are not permitted for 6 weeks after surgery.

Lateral Sesamoidectomy. The lateral sesamoid is excised through a plantar longitudinal incision. In the unusual case where the sesamoid has subluxed laterally, it can be approached through a dorsal first web space incision.

Technique

1. Under general or ankle block anesthetic and tourniquet control, the first and second metatarsal heads are palpated and their position marked on the plantar skin. A 4 cm longitudinal incision is made between these heads, extending proximally from the base of the first web space. The

subcutaneous tissue and plantar fascia are divided in line with the skin incision, and the neurovascular bundle is protected by retraction laterally (Fig. 4.6).

2. The lateral capsule of the first MTP is incised longitudinally and the plantar edge retracted. The lateral sesamoid is subperiosteally excised from its ligamentous attachments using a no. 15 scalpel. Any rents in the capsule or tears in the flexor hallucis brevis tendon are repaired with 2-0 absorbable sutures.

3. The wound is closed in layers. Care is used when approximating the edges of the plantar skin to ensure that normal skin alignment is restored so a thick scar does not form.

Postoperative Management. At discharge, the patient is instructed to remain non-weight-bearing for 3 weeks. The dressing is

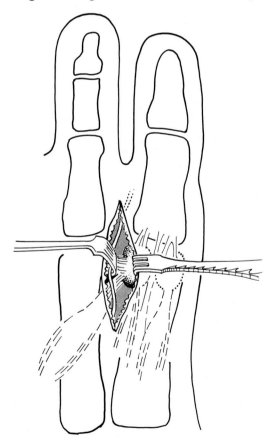

FIGURE 4.6. Plantar approach to the lateral sesamoid. The digital nerve is protected by lateral retraction.

removed at 1 week and the wound inspected. A clean sock is then worn over the foot for 2 weeks more, at which time the sutures are removed and weight-bearing is allowed in a regular shoe. Walking is gradually increased as comfortable, but running is avoided until 6 weeks after surgery.

Sesamoid Stress Fracture

As with other bones, stress fractures of the sesamoids are the result of repetitive loads that eventually cause the bones to fail. Although not common fractures, they are seen in athletes (McBryde, 1985). It is important to differentiate a stress fracture from a partite sesamoid during the radiographic evaluation.

Clinical Presentation

The athlete with a sesamoid stress fracture has slow, progressive development of pain in the ball of the foot. The pain is worsened with activities and relieved by rest. Symptoms may be present for weeks or months before the patient seeks medical care (Van Hal et al., 1982). A stress fracture may progress to osteonecrosis and osteochondritis (Irvin et al., 1985; Kliman et al., 1983).)

Physical examination reveals point tenderness to palpation directly over the involved sesamoid. Dorsiflexion of the first MTP may also be painful, particularly at the extreme. Usually there is no swelling, ecchymosis, or erythema.

Radiography

Standard AP, oblique, and lateral views of the foot should be obtained as well as an axial view of the sesamoids. Radiographs obtained early during the course of symptoms may show no abnormalities, although when repeated 3 weeks later they may demonstrate a fracture line. Partite sesamoids must be differentiated from stress fractures, which can usually be done based on the character of the line of division: A fracture is indistinct, whereas a partite sesamoid has smooth, regular edges. If the diagnosis is in doubt, the technetium bone scan readily demonstrates the fracture as a discrete area of tracer uptake.

Nonoperative Treatment

Nonoperative treatment should be attempted but often does not produce fracture union. The foot is placed in a short-leg walking cast with an extended toe plate to prevent MTP motion. A heel should be placed under the arch of the cast to transfer weight-bearing forces posteriorly. The cast is worn for 4 to 6 weeks.

If symptoms are relieved, a metatarsal pad is placed in the shoe and activities gradually increased. Patients may become asymptomatic despite overt nonunion. Should symptoms not be relieved, or if they are initially improved and then worsen, surgical excision is indicated (see Sesamoidectomy).

Sprain of First MTP Joint (Turf Toe)

Turf toe, a sprain of the plantar ligaments of the first MTP joint, occurs when the great toe is forced into hyperdorsiflexion. The term was coined as a description of a football injury associated with playing on artificial turf. In a crouched position the first MTP is dorsiflexed. Repeatedly pushing forward off the planted foot in the stance postition can damage the plantar ligaments of the first MTP joint. A more severe injury occurs when the foot is planted and another player lands on the back of first player's leg (Fig. 4.7), which forcibly dorsiflexes the first MTP joint (Coker et al.,1978; Sammarco, 1993).

The hard, unyielding character of artificial turf is a factor in the production of these injuries. Athletic participation while wearing shoes with inadequate forefoot support and cushioning is also implicated in the production of turf toe (Clanton et al., 1986; Sammarco, 1993).

Mechanism of Injury

As the first MTP joint is forcibly dorsiflexed beyond its normal arc of motion, the plantar structures tighten, causing the dorsal phalanx to impinge on the metatarsal head. If further dorsiflexion occurs, the plantar structures can stretch, tear, and finally rupture,

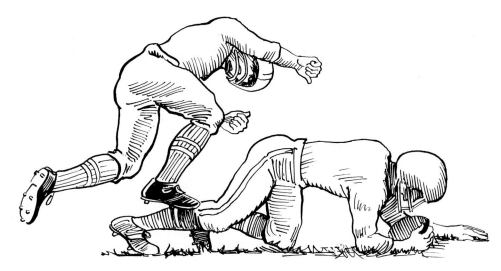

FIGURE 4.7. Hyperextension mechanism of injury due to contact.

leading to a spectrum of injuries, from sprains to frank MTP joint dislocation.

Clinical Presentation

Sprains of the first MTP joint are graded by the severity of ligamentous damage (Clanton et al., 1986). A grade I injury indicates stretching of the plantar structures. The athlete complains of plantar pain and has localized tenderness. There may be some restriction of MTP motion; swelling, if present, is slight. The athlete is usually able to continue competing with a grade I injury.

A grade II injury indicates partial tearing of the plantar ligamentous structures. There is pain and tenderness, and swelling may be noticeable on the dorsal and plantar aspects of the MTP joint. Ecchymosis may be present, and motion is limited because of guarding. The acute pain makes athletic participation impossible.

With a grade III sprain the plantar plate is completely ruptured, and there may be an associated compression fracture of the dorsal metatarsal or phalanx caused by impingement. There is significant swelling and ecchymosis, with marked restriction of motion.

Radiography

Radiographs are usually normal with all three grades of injury. Small flecks of bone may be identified adjacent to the metatarsal or phalanx with a grade III sprain, indicating capsular avulsion (Clanton et al., 1986). It is important to exclude fracture of the sesamoids (Rodeo et al., 1993). Magnetic resonance imaging (MRI) has been used to identify tearing of the plantar ligaments and may be indicated if surgery is being considered (Tewes et al., 1994).

Prevention

All athletes who perform on hard surfaces, particularly artificial turf, should wear shoes with adequate forefoot cushioning and support. The tendency to wear a lighter shoe with less support in the hope of increasing speed and improving athletic performance puts the foot at risk for developing turf toe.

Treatment

All first MTP joint sprains should be treated initially with rest, ice, compression, and elevation (RICE). A short course of oral antiinflammatory medication can help reduce pain and speed recovery. Taping provides support, primarily by blocking dorsiflexion (see Chap. 8). A shoe with the forefoot sole reinforced should be worn to limit first MTP dorsiflexion when activity resumes. Reinforcement can be provided by adding a sheet of steel or fiberglass to the sole in the forefoot. Alternatively, a semirigid insole in the shoe can provide support (Clanton et al., 1986).

Athletes with grade I injuries may be able to play with no "down time." With a grade II injury there may be a loss of up to 2 weeks of playing time, and grade III injuries may require up to 6 weeks before playing can be resumed. The consequences of an undertreated grade III injury include persistent pain, hallux valgus, and hallux rigidus (Clanton et al., 1986; Sammarco, 1993).

The only indication for surgery is removal of the intraarticularbone fragments that result from a grade III injury. These fragments may be removed through a small dorsal longitudinal incision.

First MTP Joint Dislocation

Mechanism of Injury

Dislocation of the first MTP joint results from a violent injury that forces the toe into extreme dorsiflexion. Jahss (1980) developed a classification scheme for these injuries (Fig.

4.8). Type I injury occurs when the plantar plate ruptures proximally, allowing the proximal phalanax and sesamoids to slip dorsally over the head of the metatarsal. The head is then trapped between the two tendons of the flexor hallucis brevis, fixing the toe in a dorsiflexed position.

Type II dislocations result from a greater force; there are two subtypes. With type IIA injury, there is rupture of the intersesamoid ligament, in addition to the components of a type I injury, allowing the sesamoids to splay apart. A type IIB injury includes dislocation and fracture of one of the sesamoids. If the sesamoid fracture is comminuted, the mechanism of injury must have been a crush, because pure hyperextension injuries cause the sesamoid to fail under tension with a single fracture line.

Clinical Presentation

The athlete with this injury has significant pain and swelling, and the MTP joint is held in fixed dorsiflexion. It is an uncommon injury but has been described in football and

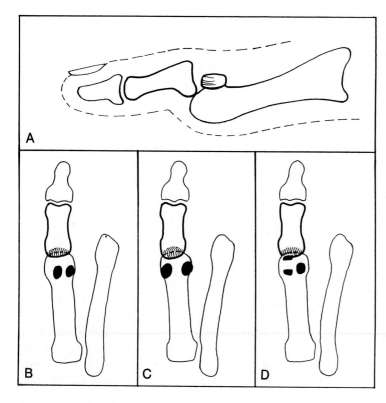

FIGURE 4.8. Dislocation of the first metatarsophalangeal joint. (A) Lateral view. (B) Type I. (C) Type IIA. (D) Type IIB.

basketball players (Clanton et al., 1986). If a player has his forefoot planted and another player lands on the back of the leg, it can cause hyperdorsiflexion of the first MTP joint, and dislocation may ensue.

Radiography

Anteroposterior, lateral, and oblique radiographs are necessary to evaluate the injury and determine its type (Fig. 4.9). The sesamoids must be carefully assessed to exclude a fracture.

Treatment

Closed reduction should be attempted first. All types can be irreducible, and therefore the injured athlete should be prepared for the possibility of open reduction. A medial or

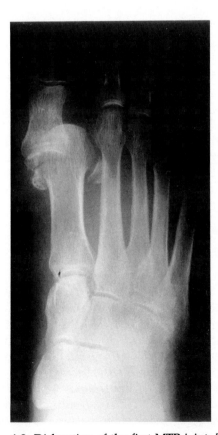

FIGURE 4.9. Dislocation of the first MTP joint. This AP radiograph shows a type IIA irreducible dislocation of the first MTP with separation of the two sesamoids.

dorsal approach is used depending on the radiographic review and the need to access medial or lateral structures in the joint (Lewis and DeLee, 1984).

Closed Reduction

Technique

1. A general anesthetic provides the best relaxation and allows a controlled reduction to be performed. A local field block about the medial forefoot or intravenous diazepam and morphine can be used in the clinic or emergency room setting.
2. The reduction maneuver begins with longitudinal traction along the great toe. The toe is brought into further hyperdorsiflexion to unlock the base of the phalanx from the head of the metatarsal. It is then brought down into normal alignment.
3. Radiographs are obtained and the position assessed. If the reduction is satisfactory and stable, immobilization is achieved by a soft bunion-type dressing that supports the great toe with tape.
4. If the reduction is unstable, a percutaneous K-wire should be inserted across the joint to maintain the position. This maneuver is performed in the operating room. After reduction of the joint, a 0.062 inch K-wire is drilled from the tip of the toe across the interphalongeal (IP) and MTP joints.
5. Radiographs are obtained to assess the reduction and the position of the implant. A soft bunion-type dressing is applied to the foot to support the great toe.

Postoperative Management. The dressing is worn for 2 weeks, and weight-bearing is allowed with a postoperative shoe. Alternatively, the reduction can be maintained with a short-leg walking cast with extension over the toes. If a K-wire has been used, it is removed at 2 weeks. At this point, a stiff-soled shoe is used for 4 weeks. Range-of-motion exercises are started to minimize stiffness at the MTP joint. Athletic activities may resume after 6 weeks, if the patient is asymptomatic. A shoe with a stiff sole under the forefoot or taping of the first MTP should be used for support during athletic activities for 3 months.

Open Reduction

Technique

1. General anesthesia or an ankle block is used. Under tourniquet control, a 4 cm longitudinal incision is centered over the medial aspect of the first MTP joint. The medial capsule is divided in line with the skin incision and the joint explored. Alternatively, a dorsal incision can be made just lateral to the extensor hallucis longus tendon.
2. Cartilage and bone fragments are removed manually and by irrigation.
3. After the joint has been reduced, a 0.062 inch K-wire is inserted longitudinally from the tip of the toe, transfixing the IP and MTP joints. The position of the implant is confirmed radiographically.
4. The wound is closed in layers and the foot wrapped with a soft bunion-type dressing to support the great toe.

Postoperative Management. Immediate weight-bearing is allowed as tolerated with a postoperative shoe and crutches. The skin sutures and pin are removed after 2 weeks. Active and passive MTP joint range of motion exercises are commenced together with therapeutic modalities including paraffin and contrast baths. A stiff-sole shoe is worn for 4 weeks. Athletic activities should be avoided for 6 weeks; when resumed, the joint should be protected by a stiff sole insert in the forefoot or taping for 3 months.

First Interphalangeal Joint Dislocation

The IP joint of the great toe can be dislocated as the result of a violent, axial loading mechanism (stubbing). It is a rare injury (Wolfe and Goodhart, 1989).

Anatomy

The first IP joint is supported medially and laterally by collateral ligaments and inferiorly by a thick plantar plate. The extensor and flexor hallucis longus tendons course the dorsal and plantar edges, respectively, to attach on the distal phalanx. As noted previously, about 15% of the population have a sesamoid associated with the IP joint that is contained in the substance of the flexor hallucis longus tendon.

Clinical Presentation

Dislocation is the result of hyperextension of the toe, which causes the distal phalanx to slip dorsally. If an IP sesamoid is present, it can become entrapped, leading to an irreducible joint. The great toe appears clawed with the tip of the toe pointing upward.

Radiography

Anteroposterior and lateral radiographs demonstrate the dislocation. Carefully review the radiographs to identify any associated fractures or entrapment of an IP sesamoid.

Treatment

Closed reduction is attempted; if satisfactory, the position is maintained by a short-leg walking cast or a soft bunion-type dressing with tape wrapped about the great toe (Jahss, 1981b). A reduction that is unstable or an irreducible dislocation requires surgical treatment. Either closed reduction and pinning or open reduction and pinning are necessary (DeLee, 1993). In cases where the sesamoid is entrapped, it should be excised (Wolfe and Goodhart, 1989).

Closed Reduction

Technique

1. A general anesthetic or a digital block with 1% lidocaine is applied. Longitudinal traction is instituted by grasping the end of the great toe. The IP joint is hyperdorsiflexed and then forced downward into the reduced position. AP and lateral radiographs are used to assess the reduction.
2. If satisfactory, the position is maintained for 2 weeks with a soft bunion-type dressing using tape to support the great toe.
3. If the joint is reducible with manipulation but the reduction is unstable, percutaneous K-wire fixation is needed. This step is

performed in the operating room under appropriate anesthesia. After reduction of the joint, a 0.062 inch K-wire is inserted from the tip of the toe, crossing the IP joint but not the MTP joint. Radiographs are obtained to assess the reduction and the position of the implant.

Postoperative Treatment. A postoperative shoe is provided with the dressing, and immediate weight-bearing is allowed. An alternative is to use a short-leg walking cast for 2 weeks, but support of the toe is not as stable with this method and the hindfoot and ankle joints are unnecessarily immobilized. Return to athletic activities is allowed after 2 weeks, using a stiff-soled shoe for an additional 4 to 6 weeks.

If pinning has been necessary, a soft dressing and postoperative shoe are used for 2 weeks. The pin is removed at 2 weeks and shoewear advanced as is possible. A stiff-soled shoe is worn for athletic activities during the next 4 to 6 weeks.

Open Reduction

Technique

1. A general anesthetic and a tourniquet are used. A transverse incision is made over the dorsum of the IP joint, and the extensor apparatus and dorsal capsule are divided. The extensor hallucis longus tendon is protected. Inspect the joint surfaces and remove any incarcerated bone fragments. If there is an interposed sesamoid, excise it.
2. After irrigating and reducing the joint, a 0.062 inch K-wire is drilled longitudinally from the tip of the toe across the joint up to (but not through) the MTP. Assess the adequacy of the reduction and position of the implant radiographically. The skin is closed with interrupted 3–0 nonabsorbable sutures, and a soft dressing is applied.
3. In the event of an open dislocation K-wire fixation is used, but the skin is left open and allowed to close secondarily. The dressing can be removed after 3 days, and wound care is instituted with regular dressing changes.

Postoperative Management. Weight-bearing is allowed with a postoperative shoe. The pin is removed at 2 weeks and shoewear advanced as allowed. A stiff-soled shoe is worn for athletic activities during the next 4 to 6 weeks.

Great Toe Phalangeal Fracture

The great toe is the second most common site of phalangeal fractures, after the fifth toe (DeLee, 1993). Fractures occur more commonly in the proximal phalanx than the distal one. The usual mechanism is a crush injury due to an object falling on the toe or another player stepping on it. Fracture can also occur if the toe is axially loaded (stubbed). With a significant crush injury the fracture can be comminuted, open, or both. If the fracture is distal, it may be associated with disruption of the nail bed. Intraarticular fractures require special consideration.

Clinical Presentation

After an acute injury to the toe, there is significant pain with weight-bearing and difficulty wearing shoes. The toe is swollen, often ecchymotic, and tender to palpation. A subungual hematoma can develop in conjunction with a distal phalangeal fracture. Lacerations or a break in the nail indicate an open fracture.

Radiography

Radiographic evaluation of the toes requires AP, oblique, and lateral views. These films allow adequate assessment of the fracture patterns as to determine appropriate treatment.

Nonoperative Treatment

Nondisplaced or minimally displaced fractures can be treated by "buddy taping" to the second toe. This maneuver allows weight-bearing in a regular shoe or a postoperative shoe depending on the level of discomfort. Taping is continued until the toe is pain-free, usually 4 weeks or less. If pain is more significant, crutches can be utilized for several days until the pain improves. An alternative is to apply a short-leg walking cast for 1 to 2 weeks. The athlete may resume activities when the toe becomes pain-free.

Severe crushing injuries can lead to long-term pain; and if the injury is intraarticular, decreased motion may be apparent and post-traumatic arthritis can develop. Most fractures, however, become painless within 4 to 6 weeks. The toe is often swollen for as long as 3 months after the injury.

Operative Treatment

Closed fractures that are severely displaced or have intraarticular displacement of more than 2 mm are treated by open reduction and K-wire fixation. If there is significant swelling, surgery can be delayed up to 7 to 10 days. Open fractures require immediate irrigation and debridement, and they are usually fixed with a K-wire, which acts as an internal splint. Closed or open fractures with a subungual hematoma should have the hematoma drained whether the fracture requires closed or open treatment.

Open Reduction

Technique

1. A general anesthesic or ankle block is used. Under tourniquet control, a 2 cm longitudinal incision is made along the medial or lateral side of the extensor hallucis longus tendon overlying the fracture.
2. After exposure, the fracture is reduced and fixed with one or two 0.062 inch K-wires, which are cut off with their ends outside the skin.
3. The wound is closed in layers, and a soft compression dressing is applied.

Postoperative Management. Weight-bearing is allowed as tolerated with a postoperative shoe. Alternatively, a short-leg walking cast may be used for 2 weeks, followed by a postoperative shoe. The sutures are removed after 2 weeks, but the postoperative shoe is worn until 6 weeks after surgery. The pins are removed at 4 to 6 weeks. At 6 weeks athletic activities can be resumed wearing a shoe with a stiff forefoot for an additional 4 weeks.

Open Phalangeal Fracture

Technique

1. A general anesthetic or ankle block is used with a tourniquet. The wound is thoroughly débrided and irrigated, using pulsatile lavage. If the fracture has significant intraarticular displacement, it is reduced and fixed as for a closed fracture. The incision used depends on the location of the fracture and the skin opening. After débriding, the wound can be extended to allow access to the displaced fracture, as needed.
2. Regardless of the degree of displacement, a K-wire is used to stabilize the toe to improve healing of the soft tissue component of the injury. A single 0.062 inch K-wire is drilled longitudinally from the tip of the toe, crossing the MTP joint.
3. The wound is allowed to close secondarily. A short-leg posterior splint is applied but is replaced after 2 days with a removable splint so wound care with dressing changes and whirlpool treatments can be undertaken. Weight-bearing is delayed until the wound has healed.
4. The K-wire is removed after 4 to 6 weeks, and unrestricted weight-bearing in a regular shoe is allowed. Athletic activities can be resumed when the wound has healed and pain is absent. A stiff forefoot shoe is used for the first 4 weeks of athletic activity.

Hallux Valgus and Bunions

Hallux valgus and bunions are among the most common deformities seen by foot specialists. A bunion is the combination of soft tissue and medial eminence of the first metatarsal that together form a medial prominence by the first MTP joint. Hallux valgus refers to lateral deviation of the great toe at the first MTP joint. These two deformities are intimately connected and may combine to cause pain with shoewear and impaired function of the first MTP joint.

Because of the high demands placed on the foot by athletes, problems with painful deformities can be significant. Athletes have shoewear considerations that may predispose to developing hallux valgus and causing bunion pain. The treatment of bunions is different for athletes and the general population.

Pathogenesis

The first metatarsal head has no muscular insertions but is stabilized by the ligaments about the first MTP joint. Valgus deviation of the proximal phalanx can cause the distal metatarsal to shift into varus. The medial capsule of the MTP joint and medial collateral ligament stretch and weaken, and the lateral side of the joint contracts. The pull of the adductor hallucis laterally translates the base of the proximal phalanx.

The lines of action of the flexor and extensor hallucis longus tendons are displaced laterally to the center of the first MTP. They then become less efficient plantarflexors and dorsiflexors, acting to further pull the toe into valgus. The first metatarsal head shifts medially, but the sesamoid apparatus remains in place, anchored by the transverse metatarsal ligament to the second metatarsal. The medial sesamoid can impinge on the cresta under the metatarsal head, and the lateral sesamoid can slip further dorsolaterally along the side of the metatarsal head. This change is accompanied by progressive pronation of the great toe.

Etiology

Hallux valgus and bunions develop as the result of an interaction between extrinsic and intrinsic factors. The most significant extrinsic factor is shoewear. It is well recognized in the general population that shoes with a narrow toebox and elevated heels worn over a period of years are associated with the development of hallux valgus and painful bunions. Other extrinsic factors include certain activities that increase lateral stress against the great toe and trauma to the first MTP joint, which alters normal joint function.

Intrinsic factors are anatomic and in some cases are determined by inheritance. They include metatarsus primus varus, a short first metatarsal relative to the second, and hyper-

mobility of the first metatarsocuneiform joint. Generalized ligamentous laxity or hyperpronation of the foot can lead to incompetence of the medial capsule of the first MTP joint, causing deformity.

Adolescents with hallux valgus have been recognized to be a population distinct from the usual patients with hallux valgus, who are most commonly middle-aged women (Coughlin, 1993a; Zimmer et al., 1989). Extrinsic factors such as shoewear are less important in young patients because their feet have not spent as much time exposed to deforming effects. Rather, intrinsic anatomic considerations have a greater role in the adolescent.

Athletes, because of their relative youthfulness, resemble the adolescent population with bunions. Factors similar to those during adolesence are important factors for causing hallux valgus in athletes. Therefore treatment of the athlete with hallux valgus is more like that for juvenile patients than for the general population.

Certain injuries are known to lead to hallux valgus. Repetitive episodes of turf toe may weaken the medial joint capsule and collateral ligament in addition to the plantar plate. Dislocation of the first MTP can also damage the medial ligaments. Excision of the medial sesamoid after a fracture predisposes to hallux valgus.

Many sports require activities that increase stress along the medial side of the forefoot, eventually causing hallux valgus. Even when participation in these sports does not lead to hallux valgus, the method of performing them may be a contributing factor (Einarsdottir et al., 1995). A pronated or abducted foot position concentrates a greater force on the medial side of the forefoot.

Sports activities that put the toe 'at risk' are varied and include squatting as a baseball catcher, crouching as a football lineman, working in the demipointe position as a ballet dancer, using skating technique as a cross-country skier, and distance running if the athlete has a pronated foot. Pushing off the planted foot produces a valgus force and occurs while serving in tennis, pitching a baseball, putting the shot, and bowling.

Shoewear also has an effect on athletes. The shoe is an important interface between the foot and its environment. A snug fit is desirable to have the most positive proprioceptive feedback, or "feel," and the most efficient energy transfer from the foot to the surface. If the shoe or boot is not properly sized, a snug fit about the midfoot and hindfoot may be accompanied by tightness in the forefoot, leading to valgus pressure on the great toe. Careful fitting is especially important for those with wide forefeet and narrow hindfeet. It is important to remember that most athletes spend most of their time in recreational shoes, and if these shoes are illfitting they can cause forefoot deformities.

Clinical Presentation

The athlete with a bunion complains of pain over the medial eminence that may be accompanied by redness and swelling. For most, symptoms occur while wearing shoes and are relieved by going barefoot. Initial treatment is to alter the shoewear so the deformity and irritated areas can be accommodated. As the problem persists, there may be pain even when the individual is barefoot or wearing shoes with a larger toebox.

Other problems can develop owing to disruption of the normal biomechanics of the joint. With contraction of the capsular ligaments that accompanies the deformity, motion of the MTP joint can be limited. Abnormal position of the sesamoids, subluxation of the phalanx laterally, pronation of the great toe, and pain combine to limit the function of the MTP joint. All of these situations can cause weakness on push-off that impairs athletic performance.

The stresses that are normally passed through the first ray may be shifted laterally, causing transfer lesions in the second and third rays: transfer metatarsalgia, intractable plantar keratoses (IPKs), stress synovitis, and hammertoe deformities (Baxter, 1994).

The physical examination determines areas of tenderness, not just in the first ray but in the whole forefoot. Any other deformities, such as hammertoes or bunionettes, and any sites of pressure buildup (IPKs, corns over

the toes) are noted. The range of motion of the first MTP joint, in particular, is important to evaluate. Pronation of the great toe should be obvious, although quantification is not practical.

Hypermobility at the first metatarsalcuneiform joint can be assessed by moving the first and second rays against each other in the dorsoplantar direction. This qualitative measurement can be performed on the opposite side and the results compared. Often this problem is noted in athletes with joint laxity who have transfer metatarsalgia.

Radiography

Radiographs of normal subjects demonstrate a valgus orientation of up to 15 degrees at the first MTP joint. Additionally, the longitudinal axes of the first two metatarsals (intermetatarsal 1–2 angle) normally diverge less than 9 degrees. These measurements are the two most important ones made from a weight-bearing AP radiograph (Fig. 4.10). Patients with a mild hallux valgus deformity have a hallux valgus angle of less than 20 degrees and an intermetatarsal 1–2 angle of less than

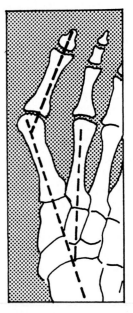

FIGURE 4.10. Hallux valgus measurements. The hallux valgus (first MTP) angle and the intermetatarsal 1–2 angle are shown.

11 degrees. The deformity is graded as moderate if the hallux valgus angle is between 20 and 35 degrees with an intermetatarsal 1–2 angle of 12 to 15 degrees. With greater angles, severe hallux valgus is present.

Other assessments are made from the radiographs. Congruency and the angulation of the joint surface are determined from the AP weight-bearing radiograph. The orientation of the articular surface of the first metatarsal head relative to the longitudinal axis of the metatarsal is termed the distal metatarsal articular angle (DMAA). The DMAA indicates the angulation of the patient's joint, which must be considered with the congruency of the joint surfaces for surgical planning (Vittetoe et al., 1994). Distal metatarsal osteotomy procedures, such as a chevron procedure, alter the DMAA but have limited effect on joint congruency (unless an adductor tenotomy is performed). Conversely, a distal soft tissue procedure such as the modified McBride technique, alters joint congruency but not the DMAA, unless combined with a proximal metatarsal osteotomy.

The hallux valgus interphalangeus angle refers to the angle between the long axes of the proximal and distal great toe phalanges. With some deformities a major component of the hallux valgus is distal to the MTP joint, which is reflected in a large hallux valgus interphalangeus angle.

The relative length of the first two metatarsals is also considered. When the second metatarsal is longer than the first, osteotomy of the first metatarsal would probably increase the disparity and can predispose to the development of transfer metatarsalgia. The position of the sesamoids relative to the metatarsal head is useful for determining medial translation of the head; and it indicates the degree of correction required to restore the normal biomechanics of the MTP joint. Radiographic evidence of arthritis—joint space narrowing, osteophytes, subchondral cysts, sclerosis—must be noted, as it influences selection of the surgical procedure.

The base of the metatarsal should also be examined, especially if there is a large intermetatarsal 1–2 angle. In some patients there is a facet on the lateral side of the proximal metatarsal shaft that articulates with the base of the second metatarsal. In these instances, the intermetatarsal angle cannot be corrected except by osteotomy of the base of the first metatarsal. The first metatarsocuneiform joint is assessed for arthritis. It is difficult to assess laxity at the joint radiographically, and the importance of the joint's orientation is unclear in regard to the genesis and treatment of hallux valgus.

Nonoperative Treatment

Nonoperative treatment must fail before surgery is contemplated. Because most patients have bunion pain when wearing shoes, changing and modifying shoewear is the mainstay of initial treatment. Proper fit is important, and refitting with a looser toebox should be attempted. As the two feet of the same individual are often of different size, it may be necessary to use different sized shoes. If this measure is unsuccessful, small pads placed around the bunion may provide adequate relief. Some shoes and boots can be modified by pressing out an area over the tender prominence.

Orthotic devices inserted into the shoe are widely prescribed for foot ailments. They may be helpful for the athlete with hallux valgus, who has pronation as a significant predisposing cause. A composite longitudinal arch support of plastizote can provide satisfactory medial support, relieving symptoms.

Operative treatment of hallux valgus and bunions can lead to restriction of first MTP joint motion. In athletes who require a large range of MTP joint motion (ballet dancers, sprinters, high jumpers) nonoperative treatment should be continued longer than would be the case for others who may not have the same demands (e.g., skiers) (Lillich and Baxter, 1986).

Operative Treatment

The symptomatic bunion that has failed an adequate course of nonoperative treatment should be considered for surgery. The preoperative evaluation of hallux valgus involves a thorough understanding of the athlete's particular deformity based on the physical examination and radiographic evaluation, as well as the demands placed on the foot by the athlete's activities. The athlete must be included in the decision-making process so as to avoid unreasonable expectations by both physician and athlete.

The high demands placed on the first MTP joint by the athlete may exceed the ability of soft tissue repairs to maintain stability. Therefore as when treating adolescent hallux valgus, it is prudent to use bone procedures, rather than soft tissue corrections alone.

Mild deformity can often be treated with a simple bunionectomy if the toe is in good alignment (Kitaoka et al., 1991). With mild or moderate deviation of the toe, a chevron bunionectomy is best (Baxter, 1994; Hattrup and Johnson, 1985; Jones et al., 1995). The modified McBride distal soft tissue procedure can be used if there is joint incongruity, but it may be associated with an increased risk of recurrence if the patient continues to place high demands on the foot.

Moderate to severe hallux valgus usually requires a modified McBride distal soft tissue procedure combined with a proximal metatarsal osteotomy to realign the first and second metatarsals (Mann and Coughlin, 1993a). In some instances of severe hallux valgus, particularly if there is MTP arthritis, it is necessary to arthrodese the MTP joint. This procedure may significantly diminish the patient's ability to participate in sports.

If there is significant hallux valgus interphalangeus, a proximal phalangeal medial closing wedge osteotomy can be added to correct this component of the deformity. Hypermobility or arthritis at the first metatarsal–cuneiform joint may require an arthrodesis of the joint.

Simple Bunionectomy

Technique

1. After anesthesia has been administered, a 4 cm medial longitudinal incision is made, centered over the bunion in the midaxial line to prevent damage to the superficial nerves. After elevating small dorsal and

plantar flaps, the medial MTP joint capsule is exposed.
2. A longitudinal incision is made in the capsule in line with the skin incision. The capsule is elevated from the medial eminence, exposing the medial sulcus.
3. A small oscillating saw is used to excise the medial eminence, beginning distally at the level of the sulcus and extending proximally in line with the first metatarsal shaft. If this cut is too shallow a beak of bone is left medially, and if it is too deep the medial metatarsal may be notched. A small rongeur or rasp is used to smooth the edges of the osteotomy.
4. Redundant medial capsule is excised, and the capsule is then closed securely with interrupted 2–0 absorbable sutures. The subcutaneous tissue is also closed with absorbable 3–0 sutures. The skin is closed with a 3–0 running nonabsorbable suture.

Postoperative Management. The foot is wrapped with a soft dressing that supports the toe, and immediate weight-bearing in a postoperative shoe is allowed. The dressing is changed at 1 week. At 2 weeks the sutures are removed, and the patient is allowed to wear a canvas tennis shoe. Passive range of motion exercises are then encouraged to maximize dorsiflexion. Power walking is allowed after 4 weeks and full return to athletic activities after 6 weeks.

Chevron Bunionectomy

Technique

1. After appropriate anesthesia and under tourniquet control a 5 cm medial longitudinal incision is made, centered over the bunion in the midaxial line to prevent damage to the superficial nerves. Small dorsal and plantar flaps are developed, and the MTP joint capsule is exposed.
2. The medial capsule is entered with an L-shaped incision. The long limb of the incision runs parallel to the skin incision in the superior third of the capsule. At the proximal end of the medial eminence the second limb of the incision runs perpendicular to the skin incision until the emi-

nence is exposed. This capsular flap is reflected plantarward, and the remaining capsule superiorly is elevated until the entire eminence and medial sulcus are free.

3. The medial eminence is removed with an oscillating saw, entering the medial eminence 1 mm medial to the sulcus and extending proximally so it exits the bone immediately behind the eminence.

4. An adductor tenotomy is made with a no. 15 blade directed through the joint while longitudinal traction is placed on the toe, distracting the joint space (Fig. 4.11A). The toe is then forced into a varus position to verify that the tenotomy is completed.

Lateral incisions or stripping of the lateral joint capsule in combination with a distal metatarsal osteotomy can devascularize the metatarsal head, leading to avascular necrosis, and so should be avoided.

5. The chevron cut is then made in the metatarsal head. The medial eminence excision leaves an exposed area of cancellous bone, and the apex of the chevron cut should be placed in the center of this cancellous bone. The oscillating saw makes the V-shaped cut with an angle of approximately 70 degrees.

6. The head fragment is separated from the shaft, translated laterally 3 to 4 mm, tipped into slight varus, and manually impacted

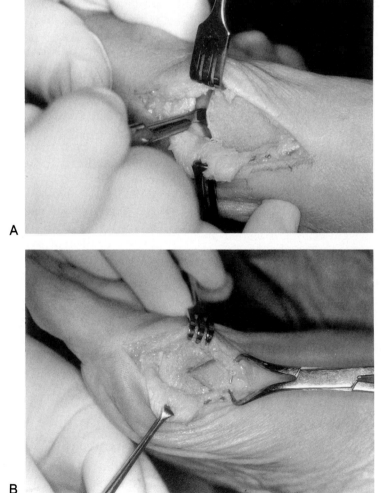

A

B

FIGURE 4.11. Chevron bunionectomy. (A) Adductor tenotomy is performed through the MTP joint with the scalpel. (B) Osteotomy with the apex in the center of the first metatarsal head.

on the metatarsal. A V-shaped shelf of distal metatarsal is left exposed medially and is cut flush with the oscillating saw so the medial border of the osteotomy is a smooth surface.

7. The osteotomy is then secured (Fig. 4.11B). If there is any question about stability, a K-wire or small fragment screw can be used to rigidly stabilize the osteotomy. Usually, however, the soft tissue closure provides adequate stability. A dorsal-to-plantar drill hole is made in the distal metatarsal shaft medially. After trimming the dorsal 2 to 3 mm of the plantar capsular flap, a no. 1 chromic suture is passed first through the drill hole and then through the plantar flap, directed inside-out and then outside in. The suture is securely tied while the toe is held in a slight varus and plantar position. This maneuver fixes the capsule, holding the metatarsal head over the sesamoids, and maintains the positioning of the osteotomy.

8. The capsule and subcutaneous layer are then closed securely with interrupted stitches of 2-O absorbable sutures, and the skin is closed with a running stitch of 3–0 nonabsorbable suture.

Postoperative Management. A soft dressing is applied to support the forefoot and great toe in the slightly overcorrected position. Ambulation with full weight-bearing is started immediately after surgery. The dressing is routinely changed at 1 week after surgery, and the foot is rewrapped with a dressing to support the toe. A second dressing change at 2 weeks allows suture removal.

A supportive dressing is usually kept in place for 3 to 4 weeks, and then a canvas tennis shoe is worn. The medial pressure on the great toe shifts it out of varus into normal alignment. Passive range-of-motion exercises are encouraged to maximize dorsiflexion. Vigorous athletic activities should be avoided until 8 to 10 weeks after surgery.

Modified McBride Bunionectomy

Technique

1. Appropriate anesthesia is administered and a tourniquet used. A 3 cm dorsal longitudinal incision is made at the base of the first web space and the adductor tendon identified at its attachment into the proximal phalanx. This tendon is released and the intermetatarsal ligament divided, taking care not to damage the closely underlying neurovascular bundle.

2. The lateral sesamoid is freed by a longitudinal incision in the first MTP joint capsule immediately superior to the lateral sesamoid. The capsule above this point is then fenestrated in multiple spots with a no. 15 blade, and the toe is gradually forced into varus, gently tearing the capsule through the fenestrations in a controlled fashion.

3. Sutures are then placed through the proximal adductor tendon, medial second MTP capsule, and lateral first MTP capsule at the level of the metatarsal head but are not tied until later.

4. A 4 cm longitudinal incision is then made over the medial eminence, and an exostectomy is performed. There are important differences in technique between this operation and a simple bunionectomy. The capsule should be entered with a V- or L-shaped incision, rather than a simple longitudinal incision, because the medial capsule must be tightened during this procedure. The osteotomy should not be made in the medial sulcus but, rather, 1 mm medial to it. If too much bone is excised medially, overcorrection producing a hallux varus may result. A small rongeur or rasp is used to smooth the edges of the osteotomy.

5. The medial capsule is tightened and imbricated, holding the toe straight on the metatarsal. The sutures in the web space are tied as pressure is placed across the forefoot against the first and fifth metatarsal heads. The wounds are closed in layers as described above.

Postoperative Management. A soft dressing is applied to support the toe, and immediate weight-bearing is allowed. The dressing is routinely changed at 1 week after surgery and the foot rewrapped with a dressing to support the toe. The sutures are removed at 2 weeks. A supportive dressing is usually kept in place for 4 to 6 weeks, and then a canvas tennis shoe is worn. Range of motion exercises are started when the dressings are removed to maximize dorsiflexion. Vigorous athletic activities should be avoided for 8 to 10 weeks after surgery.

Basilar First Metatarsal Osteotomy

The basilar first metatarsal osteotomy is added to the modified McBride distal soft tissue release if the intermetatarsal angle is more than 14 degrees. The osteotomy corrects the metatarsus primus varus component of the deformity. A basilar osteotomy should not be performed with a distal metatarsal osteotomy (e.g., a chevron bunionectomy), as the proximal and distal cuts may render the shaft nonvascular.

Technique

1. The modified McBride procedure is performed as discussed above, to the point where the medial eminence has been resected.
2. A 3 cm longitudinal incision is made over the dorsomedial base of the first metatarsal and continued medial to the extensor hallucis longus tendon down to the bone. The base of the metatarsal is exposed subperiosteally.
3. Use a crescentic saw blade to make an osteotomy 1 cm distal to the metatarsocuneiform joint. The blade is oriented such that the concavity is proximal and the long axis of the saw is perpendicular to the sole of the foot. If the axis is kept perpendicular to the metatarsal, the distal shaft elevates as it is pivoted about the osteotomy.
4. Free the osteotomy, which allows the shaft to be pivoted with lateral pressure directed against the metatarsal head. Carefully translate the metatarsal laterally; depression or elevation must be avoided.
5. Provisional fixation with a K-wire allows assessment of the position, and radiographs or fluoroscopic examination can verify satisfactory alignment. Final fixation is performed using a 3.5 mm cortical lag screw inserted from distal dorsomedial to proximal plantarlateral. The screw is countersunk, and care must be taken to prevent the dorsal cortex from cracking. An addi-

tional K-wire may be left in place to improve the initial stability of the osteotomy.
6. The modified McBride procedure then continues with closure of the medial MTP joint capsule and tightening of the sutures in the first web space, followed by closure of the wounds.

Postoperative Management. Postoperative care is similar to that used for the modified McBride procedure, except that if rigid stabilization of the osteotomy has not been achieved, protection in a short-leg walking cast for up to 4 weeks may be needed.

Proximal Phalangeal Medial Closing Wedge Osteotomy

Proximal phalangeal medial closing wedge osteotomy is a useful adjunctive procedure that can correct the hallux valgus interphalangeus component of the deformity (Fig. 4.12). When used in conjunction with a simple bunionectomy, it is referred to as the Akin procedure, a combination that has been found wanting for treatment of a standard hallux valgus deformity. However, it may be used successfully in combination with a chevron or modified McBride bunionectomy to correct a deformity distal to the MTP joint.

Technique

1. The medial longitudinal incision is extended to the interphalangeal joint of the great toe, and the proximal phalanx is exposed by subperiosteal elevation.
2. A transverse osteotomy is performed in the proximal third of the phalanx with an oscillating saw, being careful not to cut completely across the lateral cortex. A second cut is then made, starting distally 3 to 5 mm and directing the saw at an angle to the point where the first cut ended laterally, again avoiding cutting completely across the lateral cortex. This maneuver leaves a lateral hinge, which improves the stability of the osteotomy.
3. The wedge of bone (Fig. 4.12B) is removed, and a small drill point is used to make corresponding holes through the medial cortices of the proximal and distal sides of the osteotomy. A 3–0 nylon suture is passed through these holes.

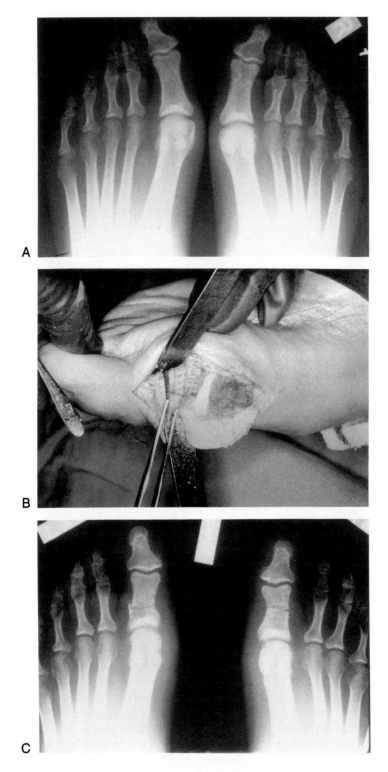

FIGURE 4.12. Akin procedure. (A) Preoperative radiographs showing the hallux valgus interphalangeus. (B) Wedge osteotomy in the first proximal phalanx, showing the segment of bone to be removed. (C) Postoperative radiograph showing the osteotomy in the first proximal phalanx.

4. The osteotomy is then closed with controlled varus pressure on the toe, and the nylon suture is securely tied. A K-wire can be inserted across the osteotomy and MTP joint if more stability is needed. Radiographs demonstrate the correction (Fig. 4.12C).
5. The wound is closed, and aftercare is performed as for the accompanying chevron or modified McBride bunionectomy.

First MTP Arthrodesis

A first MTP arthrodesis is useful for severe hallux valgus, first MTP arthritis, end-stage hallux rigidus, or as a salvage operation for a failed bunionectomy. It significantly alters the function of the first ray by converting a mobile joint to a fixed one. However, a mobile joint that is painful is less functional than a pain-free, arthrodesed joint.

Some recreational athletes can run and jump satisfactorily after arthrodesis, but all who are considering the surgery must understand that they may be trading relief of pain for a significant loss of function as a result of the procedure. Therefore the indication for the procedure in an athlete is pain unrelieved by nonoperative or other surgical means. It must be considered a salvage procedure.

Hallux Rigidus

Hallux rigidus is an affliction of the great toe MTP joint that causes limitation of motion and pain. Symptoms are similar to those caused by osteoarthritis; and although hallux rigidus may progress to arthritis, initially the joint surfaces are normal. Hallux rigidus can significantly disrupt the function of the first MTP, making athletic activities difficult. It has been recognized as a particularly disabling conditin in dancers.(Howse, 1983; Sammarco, 1982).

Etiology

The etiology of hallux rigidus is uncertain. It has been known to follow trauma to the first MTP joint, such as fracture, dislocation, or sprain (Mann and Clanton, 1988; Sammarco and Coughlin, 1993a). Other causes have

been postulated, all which increase stress across the first MTP metatarsophalangeal joint and can lead to arthitis (Mann and Haddad, 1988; Hawkins and Haddad, 1988). They include an elongated or dorsiflexed first metatarsal, osteochondritis of the first metatarsal head, and a posterior position of the sesamoids. Abnormal biomechanics caused by tightness of the plantar structures may cause impingement on the dorsal metatarsal by the base of the proximal phalanx (Fig. 4.13), leading to cartilage erosion (McMaster, 1978).

Clinical Presentation

Hallux rigidus presents as an insidious decrease in great toe motion that inhibits the ability to perform usual activities. The condition usually affects one toe, but it may be bilateral. It may occur in any age group

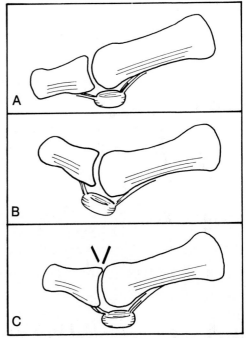

FIGURE 4.13. Hallux rigidus. (A) Relation of the metatarsal, phalanx, and sesamoid with the toe straight. (B) Normal gliding of the MTP joint during dorsiflexion pulls the sesamoid distal with the phalanx. (C) Restricted motion with hallux rigidus. Dorsal impingement occurs during attempted dorsiflexion owing to tightness of the plantar structures.

and has been described in adolescents and adults (Thompson and Mann, 1993).

Pain heralds progression of the disorder, resulting from dorsal impingement of the base of the phalanx against the metatarsal joint surface. Abnormal biomechanics convert the normal gliding of the congruent surfaces into a pinching motion at the dorsum of the joint (McMaster, 1978). This theory is supported by surgical findings of erosion of the cartilage surface about the dorsal one-third of the metatarsal head.

A dorsal prominence develops in many athletes caused by exostoses on the metatarsal head. This situation can lead to a dorsal bunion caused when the shoe rubs over the prominence and soft tissue swelling results (Fig. 4.14).

After the cartilage has been damaged, arthritis may develop, leading to further deterioration of the joint. Motion decreases, accompanied by increased pain. As the first MTP loses its normal function and dorsiflexion becomes limited, performance decreases as the gait is altered. It particularly affects toe-off, when maximum dorsiflexion is required. A decrease in push-off power affects activities as varied as running, jumping, bowling, golfing, and cross-country skiing. The forward progression of weight-bearing during stance is thrown laterally, and increased stress is placed on the second and third MTP joints, often leading to transfer metatarsalgia with pain and plantar callus formation.

Radiography

The lateral radiograph of the foot is usually diagnostic of hallux rigidus (Fig. 4.15). Early in the course of the disorder, radiographs may demonstrate a normal joint or only slight squaring of the edges of the metatarsal head on the AP view. With progression, the radiographs show osteophyte formation, first along the dorsum of the metarsal head followed by changes at the phalangeal base. The dorsal osteophyte often starts as a small point that then develops into a curving ram's horn shape. Eventually, the loss of joint space and the appearance of subchondral cysts indicates that secondary arthritis has occurred.

Nonoperative Treatment

When hallux rigidus first appears, the most common complaint is the limitation of great toe motion. Pain usually develops later. Most athletes benefit from an active and passive stretching program to maintain, and possibly increase, their existing motion. This program becomes less effective as the condition progresses.

Appropriate shoes or shoes with modifications should be selected. A stiff-soled shoe or a shoe with a fiberglass or steel sole incorpo-

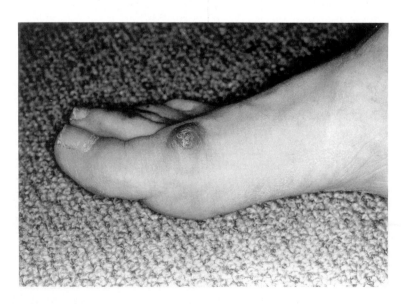

FIGURE 4.14. Hallux rigidus with a dorsal bunion. Note the prominent dorsal bunion with corn formation.

FIGURE 4.15. Hallux rigidus. Note the dorsal osteophytes off the metatarsal head and base of the proximal phalanx, which cause the dorsal bunion.

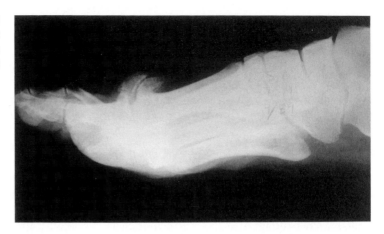

rated limits motion at the MTP joint. Obviously, it is important that the stiffened area of the shoe correspond to the MTP area. Some patients with hallux rigidus are mistakenly fit with hard, functional orthotic insoles that run from the heel to just proximal to the ball of the foot. These may aggravate symptoms because although they control the hindfoot and midfoot they permit unrestricted motion at the MTP joint.

Stiffening the sole of the shoe may eliminate pain at a cost of reduced function. A rocker bottom can be added to some sport shoes to allow a rolling action that mimics motion of the foot during stance. This modification is not feasible for many sports, however.

Significant dorsal bunions can be treated with pads or thicker socks to prevent irritation by the top of the shoe or by wearing a shoe with a higher toe box. It may be necessary to cut out the area over the prominence; with some shoes, particularly leather ones, it is possible to put a balloon patch over the prominence.

Nonsteroidal antiinflammatory medication can be helpful in eliminating pain and irritation. In most athletes, intraarticular cortisone injections are contraindicated for treatment of hallux rigidus.

Operative Treatment

Cheilectomy is the surgical procedure of choice for hallux rigidus without joint space narrowing (Mann and Clanton, 1988). This operation includes removal of osteophytes from the joint and the dorsal third of the metatarsal head joint surface, which increases motion by eliminating the site of dorsal impingement. Debulking the joint effectively loosens the joint capsule, which may help to restore congruent gliding of the joint.

If there is significant arthritis, the procedure may not be effective, and another method to treat arthritis should be employed. Such methods include resection arthroplasty (Keller procedure), implant arthroplasty, or arthrodesis, of which the latter is the only appropriate one for active individuals (Gould, 1981).

For the symptomatic joint that has become arthritic, the best option for the active patient is arthrodesis. At the expense of motion, this technique produces a first ray that is strong and can support push-off. When athletes are presented with this option, their main concern is usually how a further decrease in MTP joint motion due to the arthrodesis can be beneficial. These patients are advised that in almost all cases the arthrodesis satisfactorily relieves pain, which is the main indication for the surgery; and that when pain has been relieved, they may be able to perform activities that their present pain does not allow.

In general, although some recreational athletes may have decreased function, most have improved function after arthrodesis. It is possible to participate in running and jumping activities, such as playing basketball or volleyball, and even cross-country skiing with a first MTP joint arthrodesis.

There are various methods for performing

arthrodesis of the first MTP joint. In general, the articular surfaces of the MTP joint are removed and apposed with the toe held in a functional position. Fixation is accomplished with screws, plates, staples, or K-wires until fusion occurs.

Cheilectomy

Technique

1. A general anesthetic is administered and a thigh tourniquet applied. Alternatively, an ankle block can be administered and an Esmarch bandage used as a tourniquet at the ankle.
2. A 4 cm dorsal longitudinal incision is made over the first MTP joint, extending to the bone medial to the extensor hallucis longus tendon. The MTP joint capsule is dissected medially and laterally to expose any osteophytes on the metatarsal head or base of the phalanx. Such osteophytes are removed with a rongeur to restore the normal contour of the bones.
3. An oscillating saw or osteotome is used to remove the dorsal one-third of the metatarsal head, directing the cut from the articular surface proximally. The rongeur is used to smooth the edges of this ostectomy. It should then be possible to passively dorsiflex the MTP more than 90 degrees.
4. If there is still a block to dorsiflexion, it must be in the plantar soft tissue. Blunt dissection of the flexor brevis from the undersurface of the metatarsal may be necessary to maximize MTP dorsiflexion. However, this step may lead to postoperative fibrosis and stiffening and is not performed routinely.
5. The wound is closed in layers and a soft dressing applied.

Postoperative Management. Immediate weight-bearing is allowed in a postoperative shoe. The stitches are removed after 10 to 14 days, following which an aggressive program of dorsiflexion exercises is instituted with the assistance of a physical therapist. Athletic activities should be avoided for 6 weeks after surgery.

First MTP Arthrodesis

Technique

1. A general anesthetic or ankle block is provided and a tourniquet used. A 5 cm dorsal longitudinal incision is made over the first MTP joint medial to the extensor hallucis longus tendon. The MTP joint capsule and periosteum of both the distal metatarsal and proximal phalanx are split longitudinally and elevated medially and laterally.
2. Determining the proper alignment for the arthrodesis is critical, because it is the most significant factor for subsequent function. Most recommend fusion with the phalanx in 30 degrees of dorsiflexion and 15 degrees of valgus relative to the first metatarsal shaft. Strictly following these guidelines often leaves the tip of the toe elevated, and the great toe may rub against the second toe. The functional alignment should be determined for each foot such that the pad of the great toe just rests against a flat surface, and the toe should align itself with the long axis of the second toe. Finally, the toenail should be level, indicating proper rotational alignment of the toe.
3. When the alignment has been determined, the soft tissue at the joint is released so the toe can be positioned in its functional position. An oscillating saw is used to make parallel planar cuts, first in the metatarsal head 3 to 4 mm from the end of the bone and then in the base of the proximal phalanx. The phalangeal segment is usually firmly attached to the plantar capsule and flexor brevis tendon and must be sharply dissected free.
4. The two planar surfaces are apposed, and the position of the toe is reassessed. If further fine-tuning of the position is required, the correction is made with small cuts on the metatarsal side.
5. If present, a medial eminence is removed with the oscillating saw. A rongeur is used to smooth any sharp edges and remove osteophytes. Unless arthritic, the sesamoids are left alone.
6. *Fixation:* A 3.5 mm gliding hole is drilled from the center of the metatarsal head cut, directed proximally and laterally to just

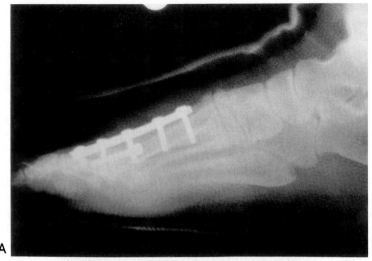

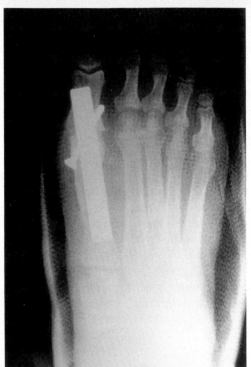

FIGURE 4.16. First MTP arthrodesis with lag screw and plate fixation. (A) Lateral view. (B) Anteroposterior view.

behind the medial eminence. Next, the toe is held in proper alignment by temporary fixation with a 0.062 inch K-wire. A 2.5 mm bit is then inserted into the proximal end of the gliding hole, and a hole is drilled into the proximal phalanx. A 3.5 mm cortical screw is inserted and tightened. A one-third tubular plate centered

over the dorsum of the MTP is used as a neutralization plate (Fig. 4.16).

7. After closing the wound in layers a soft compressive dressing is applied.

Postoperative Management. Immediate weight-bearing with a postoperative shoe is allowed. The shoe is worn for at least 6 weeks. The sutures are removed after 10 to 14 days. If there is any question about the rigidity of the construct, the foot can be protected by non-weight-bearing or a walking cast. Shoewear is routinely advanced after 6 weeks. Walking is the only activity allowed for 3 months, at which time radiographs are obtained to ensure that fusion has occurred. At that point activities can be advanced as tolerated.

Lesser Toes and Metatarsals

The lesser toes are affected by a number of injuries and deformities that can cause pain and limit athletic function. The most common site is the MTP joint. Synovitis, capsular and ligamentous tears with or without dislocation, and avascular necrosis can occur acutely or develop as the result of repetitive trauma. With injury to the MTP joint, a hammertoe may form that can cause pain in the ball of the foot or in the toe itself. Similar problems are found with clawing of multiple toes. Pain arising between the MTP joints is likely due to an interdigital neuroma. A stress fracture of the metatarsal shaft can cause pain that is perceived over the distal metatarsal.

Pressure areas can form on the plantar surfaces of the MTP joints as well as on the dorsum of the toes, particularly in the presence of a hammertoe or clawtoe deformity. The lateral fifth metatarsal head can develop a bunionette. The combination of tight shoes and bony prominences often causes corns and calluses that may be painful and limiting for the athlete.

Anatomy

The lesser metatarsal shafts have three surfaces and provide the origin of the interosseous muscles. The narrow metatarsal neck flares into medial and lateral tubercles for attachment of the collateral ligaments. The metatarsal heads have condyloid articular surfaces that extend more plantarward than dorsally.

The great toe has two phalanges and one IP joint, whereas there are three phalanges and

two IP joints in each of the four lesser toes. The proximal phalanx has a large base with an oval articular surface and a flat head with a trochlear articular surface. The middle phalanx is shorter, and the distal phalanx is quite small. Both of the distal phalanges have trochlear articular surfaces. The primary motion of the MTP joint is dorsiflexion, whereas the proximal interphalangeal (PIP) and distal interphalangeal (DIP) joints primarily plantarflex.

The lesser toe MTP joints are stabilized by strong ligaments (Johnston et al., 1994). The fibrocartilaginous plantar plate is attached to the base of the proximal phalanx and is the strongest supportive structure. Proximally it attaches to the metatarsal through the collateral and suspensory glenoid ligaments. On either side are attachments to the intermetatarsal ligaments, and on the plantar aspect are attachments to the flexor digitorum longus tendon sheath and fibers of the plantar aponeurosis.

The IP joints are supported by collateral ligaments that extend from the head of one phalanx to the base of the next (Sarrafian, 1983). Plantar plates are also present at the IP joints and have attachments underneath for the long flexor tendon sheath.

The extrinsic muscles are located in the leg, with the extensors innervated by branches of the peroneal nerve and the flexors innervated by the posterior tibial nerve. The intrinsic muscles of the foot are innervated by the medial and lateral plantar branches of the posterior tibial nerve. The flexor digitorum longus acts through its tendinous attachment onto the distal phalanx. The flexor digitorum brevis tendons split into two slips at the level of the proximal phalanx, and the long flexor passes between them. They run together until the middle phalanx where the short flexor tendons attach to the plantar surface.

The extensor digitorum longus tendon joins with the corresponding tendon of the extensor digitorum brevis for toes 2, 3, and 4 at the level of the MTP joint, and both insert into the extensor hood overlying the proximal phalanx (Couglin, 1993; Sarrafian and Topouzian, 1969). A central slip extends distally and attaches to the dorsum of the middle phalanx, and two lateral slips extend farther, converging to attach to the distal phalanx. The extensor hood is anchored proximally on both sides to the transverse intermetatarsal ligaments and plantar plate through the extensor sling. The fifth toe does not have an extensor brevis tendon and has an atrophic extensor hood.

The four dorsal interosseous muscles arise from the shafts of metatarsals 2 to 5 and abduct the toes relative to the axis of the second ray (Sarrafian, 1983). The three plantar interossei arise from metatarsals 3, 4, and 5 and are toe adductors. The four lumbricals arise from the medial side of the long flexor tendons to the lesser toes and attach into the medial portion of the respective extensor hood.

Extension of the MTP joint occurs through action of the long extensor on the sling mechanism of the extensor hood (Sarrafian and Topouzian, 1969). The PIP is extended by the central slip of the long extensor, and the DIP is extended by the terminal extension of this tendon onto the distal phalanx.

The interossei and lumbrical muscles act to plantarflex the MTP joints because their tendons pass plantar to the axis of rotation of these joints (Sarrafian, 1983). The lumbrical also acts to extend the IP joints through its insertion into the extensor hood. The PIP is flexed by the short flexor and the DIP by the long flexor.

The medial and lateral plantar branches of the posterior tibial nerve originate in the tarsal tunnel and pass into the foot, where they provide motor branches to the intrinsic muscles and sensory branches to the plantar aspect of the foot. The medial division supplies the area under the first three rays and the tibial side of the fourth, with the remaining area innervated by the lateral branch.

The common plantar digital nerves are the terminal sensory branches of these nerves and travel in the interval between the plantar aponeurosis and the deeper flexor digitorum brevis tendons; they extend distally. Each nerve enters the interosseous space just proximal to the metatarsal head and lies superficial to the intermetatarsal ligament. At this level the nerve divides into digital branches for each side of the corresponding web space.

Metatarsophalangeal Joint Chronic Conditions

Sprains and Synovitis

The plantar plate is the primary plantar stabilizer of the MTP joint (Coughlin, 1989, 1993b; Myerson and Shereff, 1989; Smith and Reischl, 1988). Injury occurs after a misstep or abrupt landing on the ball of the foot, causing forced dorsiflexion of the toe. The joint becomes irritated, and synovitis develops. The athlete can usually recall a particular traumatic episode.

Chronic irritation can also lead to synovitis, occurring most commonly in the second MTP joint (Coughlin, 1989, 1993b; Smith and Reischl, 1988). The second metatarsal is the longest and in many people extends distal to the first metatarsal. During toe-off at the end of stance, the second MTP joint may be chronically stressed, causing attritional damage to the plantar plate. Other factors can lead to a transfer of weight-bearing through the second ray, including altered biomechanics of the first MTP joint.

Clinical Presentation

The athlete is able to localize the pain to the ball of the foot and describes weight-bearing as uncomfortable. The toe and ball of the foot usually appear normal with no evident swelling or bruising. The MTP joint on the plantar aspect of the foot can be pinched between the examiner's thumb and the second or third finger dorsally. Tenderness with the manuever identifies this point as the site of pain. It is important to similarly palpate the adjacent MTP joints and then the intermetatarsal spaces to confirm the site of maximum tenderness.

The stability of the MTP joint can be assessed qualitatively. Stabilize the distal metatarsal with one hand, and while grasping the proximal phalanx with the other attempt to move them against each other in a dorsoplantar direction (Fig. 4.17). This test has been designated the drawer test (Thompson and Hamilton, 1987). The manuever is also uncomfortable in an athlete with MTP synovitis.

The interspaces about the MTP joint should be carefully palpated to ensure that the pain is not coming from an interdigital neuroma. The first MTP joint biomechanics are assessed to determine if an abnormality is causing a transfer metatarsalgia (Coughlin, 1993b).

Radiography

Routine radiographs including an AP, lateral, and oblique views are necessary to exclude a fracture. Otherwise, in most patients with synovitis or a sprain the radiographs are unremarkable. The first MTP joint should be evaluated and the relative lengths of the first and second metatarsals assessed to determine if a short first ray may be contributing to the lesser MTP problem through a transfer metatarsalgia mechanism.

Nonoperative Treatment

Most athletes can be treated successfully with a combination of activity limitation and oral antiinflammatory medications. A stiff insole placed under the MTP joint limits motion and allows continuation of activities. Taping the toe with a loop over the dorsum of the proximal phalanx also stabilizes the toe (Coughlin, 1993b). A toe crest is a stabilizing device with an elastic loop that fits over the proximal phalanx and can provide support.

HAPADS are a simple treatment that can decrease the weight-bearing stress at the MTP joint (Holmes and Timmerman, 1990). They are felt pads with an adhesive backing that are placed in the shoe just proximal to the MTP joint, resting on the insole. The athlete positions and adjusts them to obtain optimal relief.

HAPAD Placement

1. The athlete is instructed to make a mark on the point of maximal tenderness on the ball of the foot with lipstick and then to step barefoot into the shoe. The lipstick marks the insole at the corresponding spot and indicates proper placement of the HAPAD. The pad is triangular and should be placed on the insole with the broad base located just proximal to the mark.
2. The athlete is instructed to remove only a small section of the covering over the adhesive initially, just enough to prevent it from slipping. The patient then wears the shoe for a few hours to determine if the pad is in the correct position. It can be moved about to obtain satisfactory placement.
3. The entire covering is then removed from the adhesive, and the HAPAD is fixed into this position. The pad effectively transfers the forces of weight-bearing proximal to the MTP joint.

Hard orthotics that support the arch may increase the stress on the MTP joint if they end just proximal to the ball of the foot, and their use should be discontinued during the treatment phase for this problem.

Injection of corticosteroid should be withheld except for the most recalcitrant cases because of the possibility of weakening already irritated ligaments and inducing subluxation or dislocation of the joint. Steroid

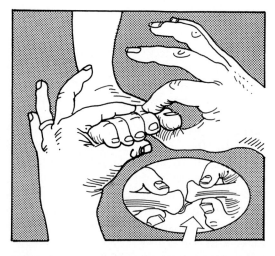

Figure 4.17. Drawer test. Instability of the second MTP joint is demonstrated with the drawer test. Dorsal subluxation of the phalanx against the stabilized metatarsal is demonstrated.

injection should be used only after other treatment has failed to provide relief and the alternative treatment would be surgery. Should the steroid injection cause ligament rupture, it is treated surgically.

Steroid Injection

1. Injection of corticosteroid is done using a 25 gauge needle. A mixture 1 ml of 1.0% lidocaine and 0.5% bupivacaine (Marcaine) both without epinephrine, in a 1 ml aliquot is partially infiltrated into the skin, and the needle is then directed into the joint.
2. When the joint has been entered, the needle is left in place while the syringe is disconnected and a second syringe with only 1 ml of corticosteroid is attached. Usually 0.3 ml of the steroid is injected into the joint. The syringe with the local anesthetic is then replaced on the needle, and while continuing to gently infiltrate the local anesthetic the needle is withdrawn. This method ensures that the steroid is injected only into the joint, and that none is leaked into the subcutaneous tissue where it may damage the fat or subcutaneous tissue.
3. The effect of the local anesthetic in the joint is experienced for several hours. It should block pain coming from the joint— but only from the joint. Therefore this therapeutic injection can also be used to confirm the diagnosis. If there is pain coming from any adjacent structures, which would not have been blocked by this injection, they can be identified separately from the MTP joint.

Operative Treatment

Surgery is indicated when deformity has occurred, the MTP is dislocated, or the pain cannot be managed with nonoperative methods. A simple synovectomy can be performed if there is no deformity or instability at the MTP joint. Otherwise, a flexor-to-extensor tendon transfer or collateral ligament repair should also be added. Coughlin (1993b) reported 71% good to excellent results after combined synovectomy and tendon transfer in athletic patients.

Synovectomy

Technique

1. Synovectomy of the lesser MTP joints is performed as an outpatient procedure with a local or general anesthetic. An S-shaped incision of approximately 2 cm is made over the dorsum of the MTP joint. A straight longitudinal incision should not be used because it may cause a scar that can contract and limit motion of the joint.
2. The extensor tendons are retracted to the side, and the joint capsule is opened transversely. With distraction on the toe the joint can be opened and a small rongeur used to débride the synovium.
3. The MTP joint capsule is approximated with 3–0 absorbable suture, and the subcutaneous layer and skin are closed separately.

Postoperative Management. The foot is dressed, and weight-bearing is allowed immediately with a postoperative shoe. The sutures are removed at 10 to 14 days, and shoewear is advanced. At first, only walking is allowed; after 2 weeks, however, full return to activities may begin.

Subluxation and Dislocation

If the MTP is more severely injured there may be rupture of the collateral ligaments or the plantar plate. If so, the joint is destabilized, and the action of the long tendons on the toe can cause the MTP joint to subluxate or dislocate (Coughlin, 1989, 1993b; Myerson and Shereff, 1989). It can occur acutely or develop as the result of recurrent or repetitive trauma to the forefoot (Smith and Reischl, 1988).

Clinical Presentation

With an acute injury there is significant swelling sometimes accompanied by bruising. If a collateral ligament is torn, the toe deviates away from the side of the torn ligament (Fig. 4.18), and there appears to be splaying between it and the adjacent toe. If the plantar plate has ruptured, the toe can dislocate dorsally. It may seen to be in proper

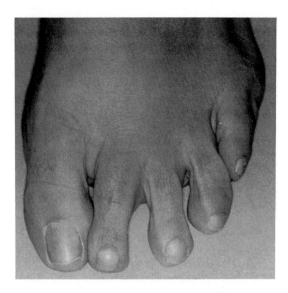

FIGURE 4.18. Metatarsophalangeal collateral ligament injury. Rupture of the lateral collateral ligament of the second MTP results in splaying between the second and third toes.

alignment, but an elevated attitude appears with weight-bearing. Again there is swelling of the ball of the foot and possibly bruising. As the dorsally dislocated proximal phalanx slips over the top of the metatarsal head, the head is depressed, which may appear as a prominence on the plantar surface. Later, as the swelling decreases it may be possible to manually relocate and dislocate the MTP with the drawer test (Thompson and Hamilton, 1987). In instances where the metatarsal head is caught between slips of the flexor tendon or plantar plate, the joint may be irreducible.

Radiography

At a minimum, AP and lateral radiographs must be taken to identify the deformity and to ensure that there has not been a concomitant fracture. The lateral radiograph may be difficult to interpret owing to overlapping views of all the MTP joints. If subluxation is present, the AP view may show the joint to be incongruent, or the toe may be obviously deviated to one side.

With a frank dislocation the AP radiograph shows loss of the MTP joint with overlap of the phalangeal base and metatarsal head.

There may be lateral displacement of the phalanx on the metatarsal.

Nonoperative Treatment

Rest, ice, elevation, and compression (RICE) comprise the appropriate treatment for subluxation if there is significant swelling. A toe crest or toe taping in a reduced position can maintain alignment. Subsequently, HAPADs are used to transfer weight-bearing stress proximally.

Operative Treatment

An acutely dislocated toe should be treated immediately. Closed reduction under a 1% lidocaine digital block is usually successful. If there has been soft tissue interposition, delay in treatment, or significant swelling, closed reduction may not be possible or may be unstable. In these cases an open reduction with percutaneous K-wire fixation is performed.

If the dislocation is long-standing or there has been significant trauma to the soft tissue, it may be impossible to maintain the reduction even with pin fixation. A Girdlestone-Taylor flexor-to-extensor tendon transfer is then used to provide stability (Barbari and Brevig, 1984; Coughlin, 1993b).

Rupture of a collateral ligament with deviation of the toe is treated by primary repair of the ligament. With severe damage or a long-standing deformity, a combination of Girdlestone-Taylor tendon transfer and release of the tight structures on the opposite side of the rupture is used.

Closed Reduction

1. To perform a closed reduction, a digital block with a 25 gauge needle and 3 ml of local anesthetic is used. The latter is injected just proximal to the MTP joint on both sides, both superficially and deep to block both dorsal and plantar digital nerve branches on either side of the MTP joint.
2. The toe is then grasped, with longitudinal traction applied with one hand while the other hand manipulates the proximal phalanx back into a reduced position.

3. The reduction is maintained by taping over the dorsum of the proximal phalanx. A postoperative shoe or other flat shoe should be worn for 2 weeks. Shoewear can be advanced.

Open Reduction. Dorsal dislocation of an MTP joint that cannot be reduced closed is treated by open reduction.

Technique

1. Appropriate anesthesia is provided, and a tourniquet is used. The joint is approached through a 2 cm S-shaped incision centered over the MTP.
2. After retracting the extensor tendons, a transverse dorsal capsulotomy is made and the joint opened. Reduction is performed, with longitudinal traction applied through the toe.
3. The joint is distracted and inspected for damage to the articular surface; loose bone fragments within the joint may result from marginal fractures at the time of injury. Such fragments should be extricated mechanically or by irrigation.
4. If the joint appears stable, the wound can be closed. If there is any concern about stability the reduction is maintained with a 0.062 inch K-wire, which is inserted from the tip of the toe through the phalanges and across the MTP joint. The pin is left protruding 5 mm through the skin so that it can be subsequently removed.
5. In cases where the MTP joint has been dorsally dislocated for an extended time, the surrounding soft tissue may shorten, having adapted to the dislocated position. It may be necessary to perform Z-lengthening of the extensor tendons to accomplish reduction. Maintaining the reduction may also be difficult and require stabilization other than a temporary K-wire. The Girdlestone-Taylor flexor-to-extensor transfer can be added to provide additional stability.
6. After closure of the wound in layers, a soft dressing is applied.

Postoperative Management. Immediate weight-bearing is allowed with a postoperative shoe. The skin sutures are removed after 7 to 10 days, and the pin is removed after 2 weeks. A regular shoe is then worn, with activities advanced until they are full and complete by 4 weeks.

Girdlestone-Taylor Tendon Transfer

Technique. The technique is shown in Figure 4.19.

1. A general anesthetic and a thigh tourniquet are used. A calf tourniquet or Esmarch bandage at the ankle tends to preferentially squeeze the long flexor muscles of the calf and causes the toes to rest in a clawed position. It is then difficult to properly adjust the tension on the tendon transfer to align the toe.
2. The MTP joint is exposed through a dorsal 2 cm S-shaped incision. The distal limb of the incision extends onto the midproximal phalanx, and the periosteum is exposed.
3. A second incision is made on the plantar aspect of the toe longitudinally from the distal flexion crease to 1 cm proximally. Immediately below the skin the flexor tendon sheath is opened for the length of the wound. The flexor digitorum longus tendon, which runs between the two limbs of the brevis tendon, is grasped with a small mosquito clamp and cut distally from its insertion on the distal phalanx with a #11 scalpel (Fig. 4.20).
4. The flexor digitorum longus tendon has a medial raphe separating its two halves. It is split distally with the scalpel, and with small clamps placed on the two halves it is separated by pulling them apart.
5. A small, curved clamp is tunneled against the bone of the proximal phalanx from the proximal incision to the distal one along one side. One of the separated limbs of the flexor longus tendon is grasped by the curved clamp and pulled through to the dorsal wound. The other limb is similarly pulled up along the opposite side.
6. After reducing the MTP joint and maintaning it with a longitudinal K-wire, the two limbs of the flexor tendon are sutured together over the top of the proximal phalanx with 2–0 absorbable suture.
7. The wounds are closed in layers, and a soft dressing is applied.

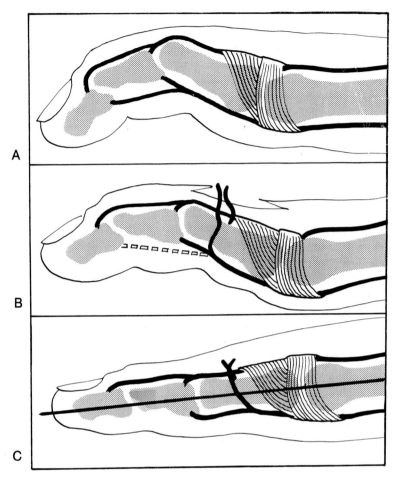

FIGURE 4.19. Girdlestone-Taylor flexor-to-extensor tendon transfer. (A) Pathologic toe with dorsiflexion at the MTP joint and flexion at the PIP and DIP joints. The flexor (dorsal) and extensor (plantar) tendons are indicated, as is the extensor sling apparatus. (B) Long flexor has been released from its attachment at the distal phalanx, split, and each half routed along one side of the proximal phalanx through to the dorsal wound. (C) Toe is held straight by the transferred long flexor tendon, whose two halves have been sewn together over the proximal phalanx. K-wire provides temporary fixation.

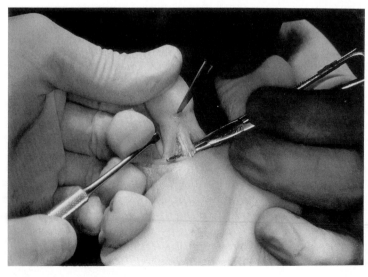

FIGURE 4.20. Girdlestone-Taylor flexor-to-extensor tendon transfer. The long flexor tendon is exposed and divided off the base of the distal phalanx.

Postoperative Management. Immediate weight-bearing is allowed with a postoperative shoe. The K-wire is kept in place for 2 to 3 weeks and then removed. Advancement to a regular shoe and active range-of-motion exercises are started. Athletic activities should be deferred for 6 weeks after this point, and a shoe with a stiffened forefoot should be used for three additional months to protect the repair.

Collateral Ligament Repair

Technique

1. A general anesthetic is provided and a thigh tourniquet used. A 3 cm dorsal longitudinal incision is made in the web space on the side of the ligament tear (between the splayed toes).
2. The lateral joint capsule and collateral ligament are contiguous structures and are repaired together. A vertical elliptical incision is made through the joint capsule and collateral ligament at the level of the MTP joint. An ellipse of tissue of dimensions 1.0 × 0.5 cm is removed.
3. Two or three sutures of absorbable 3–0 are placed in simple, interrupted fashion but not tied.
4. A longitudinal 0.062 inch K-wire is drilled to immobilize the MTP joint in neutral. The sutures are then tied, and the wound is closed in layers with a soft dressing applied.

Postoperative Management. Weight-bearing is allowed with a postoperative shoe. The skin sutures and K-wire are removed after 2 weeks. Walking in a regular shoe is allowed, and athletic activities are advanced 3 to 4 weeks after surgery.

Freiberg's Infraction

Freiberg's infraction is an osteochondrosis of the metatarsal head, most commonly involving the second metatarsal but also seen in the third and fourth metatarsals (Katcherian, 1994). The exact etiology is unknown, but an assumed insult causes avascular necrosis in the metatarsal head, leading to collapse of the subchondral bone, deformity of the MTP joint, and finally arthritis. It has been suggested that trauma, as a single event or repetitive, is the insult. The second metatarsal epiphysis is most vulnerable to trauma during the early teen years, and it has been proposed that microfractures caused by abnormal stress and bone fatigue leads to the avascular necrosis (Braddock, 1959; Douglas and Rang, 1981; Helal and Gibb, 1987; Katcherian, 1994). A mechanism of dorsal impingement due to incongruent joint movement during dorsiflexion, similar to that seen with hallux rigidus, has been proposed to explain the traumatic insult (Helal and Gibb, 1987; Katcherian, 1994; McMaster, 1978). A primary vascular deficiency may predispose to the development of osteochondrosis (Wiley and Thurston, 1981).

Clinical Presentation

Freiberg's infraction occurs predominantly in females and usually appears during the early teenage years. The first symptom is pain in the ball of the foot with weight-bearing (Helal and Gibb, 1987; Katcherian, 1994). It is worse with activities that require excessive dorsiflexion of the toes, and the athlete may complain of limitation of motion in the involved toe.

There is tenderness to palpation of the involved MTP joint. There may be limitation of dorsiflexion and pain with passive dorsiflexion. Swelling may develop secondary to MTP joint synovitis.

Radiography

Radiographs obtained at the onset of symptoms may be negative, but subsequent studies show a lucent crescent in the subchondral bone of the metatarsal head. A bone scan at this point shows increased uptake at the involved metatarsal head.

Over time there may be progression, characterized by collapse of the subchondral bone with flattening of the metatarsal head seen on an AP radiograph (Fig. 4.21). Later osteophytes may form about the deformed metatarsal head, and secondary adaptations are found on the base of the proximal phalanx as the joint becomes frankly arthritic.

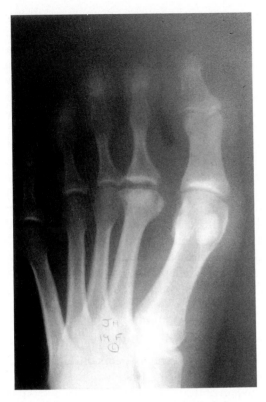

FIGURE 4.21. Freiberg's infraction. This radiograph shows flattening of the second metatarsal head with a crescent sign.

Several radiographic staging schemes have been proposed, but they do not correlate with prognosis or the patient's symptoms (Katcherian, 1994; Smilie, 1957; Thompson and Hamilton, 1987).

Nonoperative Treatment

Nonoperative treatment should be used first in all cases; and when started early it may prevent subchondral bone collapse in the metatarsal head and the development of arthritis. During episodes of pain, a short-leg walking cast or strict non-weight-bearing may relieve symptoms.

After this initial treatment the MTP joint is protected with a HAPAD or similar permanent metatarsal pad built into the insole of the shoe. A stiffened forefoot or rockerbottom sole is used to decrease motion at the MTP joint. Elevated heels should be avoided, as they tend to increase stress at the MTP joint.

If the joint has a normal shape, prevention of collapse is the prime concern. Activity should be restricted if pain cannot be relieved with shoe modifications. If collapse has already occurred, activity restrictions and oral antiinflammatory medications can be used for episodes of pain.

Operative Treatment

If osteophytes have formed and are limiting MTP motion, a cheilectomy and joint débridement can be performed to eliminate the mechanical block (Katcherian, 1994; Mann and Coughlin, 1993b). When cartilage has been significantly affected or arthritis has developed, a DuVries metatarsal head arthroplasty with or without volar plate interposition has been recommended (Lavery and Harkless, 1992). Removal of the entire metatarsal head alters weight-bearing across the forefoot and can lead to intractable plantarkeratoses under the adjacent metatarsal heads. A dorsiflexion osteotomy of the metatarsal neck to elevate the head and rotate the more normal plantar joint surface against the proximal phalanx was proposed by Gauthier and Elbaz (1979) and modified by Kinnard and Lirette (1989).

Cheilectomy

Technique

1. A general anesthetic is provided and a thigh tourniquet used, or an ankle block can be applied with an Esmarch bandage at the ankle as a tourniquet. The joint is approached through a dorsal S-shaped incision and the extensor tendon is retracted or Z-lengthened.
2. A dorsal MTP joint capsulotomy is performed, and the metatarsal head and base of the proximal phalanx are exposed subperiosteally medially and laterally.
3. A small rongeur removes osteophytes and contours the head to a normal shape. The toe is moved through a range of motion to ensure that there is no remaining mechanical block at the end of the procedure.
4. The cartilage on the phalangeal base and metatarsal head is left intact. If it has been

significantly damaged, a DuVries or inter-position arthroplasty is performed.

5. The wounds are closed in layers, and a soft dressing is applied.

Postoperative Management. Immediate weight-bearing is allowed with a postoperative shoe. The sutures are removed at 10 to 14 days, and active and passive range of motion exercises are started. Shoewear is also advanced. Athletic activities may be resumed after 3 to 4 weeks.

Dorsiflexion Osteotomy of Metatarsal Neck

Technique

1. A general anesthetic is provided and a thigh tourniquet used, or an ankle block can be applied with an Esmarch bandage at the ankle as a tourniquet. The joint is approached through a dorsal S-shaped incision, and the extensor tendon is retracted or Z-lengthened.
2. A dorsal MTP capsulotomy is performed and the metatarsal head and base of the proximal phalanx are exposed subperiosteally medially and laterally.
3. A small rongeur removes osteophytes and contours the head to a normal shape.
4. A closed dorsal wedge osteotomy is then made in the head and neck (Fig. 4.22). The proximal cut is made where the neck meets the metatarsal head so it is perpendicular to the long axis of the metatarsal. The distal cut is made in the center of the defect

in the metatarsal head, directed proximally and inferiorly, at a 45 degree angle to the sole of the foot.

5. The head fragment is then rotated over the end of the metatarsal neck. A 0.062 inch K-wire is used as a drill point to make transverse holes in the dorsal head and metatarsal. A single loop of 2-0 absorbable suture is passed through the holes to stabilize the head fragment.
6. After closure a short-leg walking cast is applied.

Postoperative Management. Weight-bearing is allowed after 3 to 5 days. The cast is removed after 3 weeks, and a postoperative shoe worn for 3 weeks more. Activities are then advanced as tolerated.

Hammertoes and Clawtoes

Hammertoes and clawtoes are common forefoot deformities in the general population (Fig. 4.23). Their appearance and the disability they can cause have been well documented in a range of athletes, including runners, dancers, and basketball players (Lutter, 1982; McDermott, 1993; Sammarco, 1982).

The terms hammertoe and clawtoe are often used imprecisely to describe similar common deformities that occur in the lesser toes. According to Myerson and Shereff (1989), both have extension at the MTP joint and plantarflexion at the PIP joint. The clawtoe also has a flexed posture at the DIP

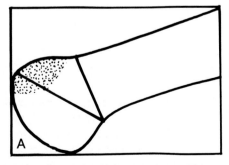 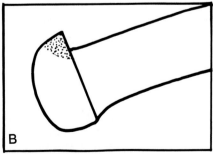

FIGURE 4.22. Dorsiflexion osteotomy of the metatarsal head for Freiberg's infraction. (A) The two limbs of the osteotomy are indicated, as is the dorsal wedge to be removed that includes most of the pathologic bone (stippled). (B) Closure of the osteotomy elevates the metatarsal head and shortens the metatarsal.

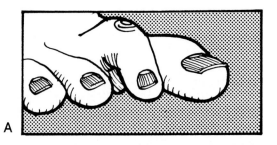

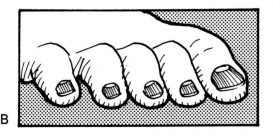

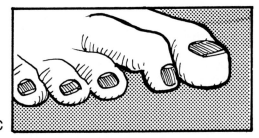

FIGURE 4.23. Hammertoe, clawtoes, and mallet toe deformities. (A) Hammertoe deformity. (B) Multiple clawtoes. (C) Mallet toe deformity.

joint, whereas the hammertoe is straight or extended. Coughlin and Mann (1993) stated that although both deformities have flexion at the PIP joint, the hammertoe has extension at the MTP, and the clawtoe does not. The differences between these definitions are probably not important clinically. A scheme is offered that provides direction about the management of these deformities based on the site of pathology.

Pathogenesis

Hammertoes and clawtoes develop as the result of several mechanisms that include imbalance between the extrinsic and intrinsic muscles, the effects of trauma, restrictive shoewear, and incompetence of the ligaments about the toe. As a generalization, a hammertoe can be considered to be caused

by a problem intrinsic to that toe, whereas a clawtoe is the result of pathology acting on the toe from a distance.

By this definition, when the pathology is rupture of the plantar plate and loss of support about the MTP joint, the deformity that results is a hammertoe. It can be caused by trauma, in which case there is usually only one toe involved, (though there may be more) or by a disease process such as rheumatoid arthritis that damages many MTP joints (Rau and Manoli, 1991). The pathology is still in the the MTP joint.

Wearing shoes with a short toebox may encourage the development of a hammertoe. If there is inadequate room for the toe to rest fully extended, it effectively shortens by flexion of the MTP and PIP joints, taking the attitude of a hammertoe. The plantar plate of the MTP joint is stretched and, over time, may become incompetent. There may also be secondary contracture of the collateral ligaments and dorsal structures about the MTP joint that adapt to the hammered position.

Clawtoe deformities are usually multiple because the same extrinsic process affects multiple toes (Barbari and Brevig, 1984). Clawtoes are manifestations of an imbalance between the extrinsic muscles of the leg and the intrinsic muscles of the foot. When the extrinsic muscles overpower the intrinsic muscles, a clawed toe results. Intrinsic weakness is seen with diabetic neuropathy, compartment syndrome in the foot, or the result of prolonged casting that leads to intrinsic wasting. Clawtoes (Fig. 4.24) may result from neuromuscular disorders, such as Charcot-Marie-Tooth disease, and are associated with the cavus foot, whether congenital or acquired.

Clinical Presentation

The abnormal anatomy of hammertoes and clawtoes leads to several problems. The elevated PIP joint can rub against the top of the shoe, causing pain, a corn (Fig. 4.25), or an ulcer. The end of the toe may strike the sole of the shoe, causing a painful "end" corn. With dorsiflexion at the MTP joint, pain and pressure problems can develop under the ball

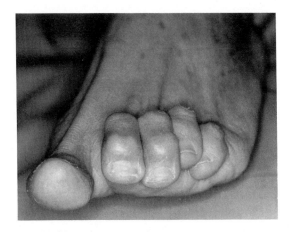

FIGURE 4.24. Clawtoes. There is clawing of all four lesser toes.

of the foot. A single hammertoe may have a discrete callus under it, termed an intractable plantar keratosis (IPK).

Clawtoes are usually associated with more diffuse callus formation. As all of the toes dorsiflex, not only are the metatarsal heads depressed but the normal fat pad under the ball of the foot is drawn distally. This loss of the normal cushioning under the metatarsal heads can lead to pain and forefoot fatigue.

It is important to differentiate between flexible and fixed deformities when considering treatment. Both hammertoes and clawtoes start out flexible, meaning that they can be passively corrected. Later the soft tissues about the joints adapt to the abnormal position, and these entities are now considered to be fixed deformities.

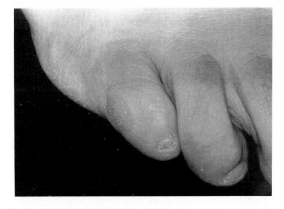

FIGURE 4.25. Hammered fifth toe with a dorsal corn.

Nonoperative Treatment

A flexible hammertoe can usually be treated by depressing the proximal phalanx. A toe crest has an elastic loop that fits over the base of the toe, depressing the proximal phalanx. The same effect can be obtained with a loop of tape placed over the toe and anchored to the ball of the foot. Shoes must have an adequate toebox so the toe can fully extend and not cause rubbing against the dorsum of the PIP joint. If an IPK has formed under the MTP joint, a HAPAD or insole with a metatarsal pad placed just proximal to the MTP can relieve the pressure there. Moleskin or sponge pads can be placed over the PIP or end of the toe to relieve corns.

Rigid hammertoes and clawtoes cannot be treated with toe crests or taping. A HAPAD may help relieve pain in or under the MTP joint of a rigid hammertoe. Clawtoes usually require a metatarsal pad across the entire forefoot to relieve the weight on the ball of the foot. Shoe accommodations to provide a toebox with more room and pads to treat corns can be useful.

Operative Treatment

A hammertoe that is flexible can be treated with a Girdlestone-Taylor flexor to extensor tendon transfer to rebalance the soft tissues (Coughlin, 1993b). The deforming force of the long flexor tendon that acts on the PIP is released and converted to a conforming force to depress the proximal phalanx and support the MTP joint. Multiple Girdlestone-Taylor procedures can be used to correct clawtoes that are flexible (Barbari and Brevig, 1984).

Rigid hammertoe or clawtoe deformities require bone resection at the PIP joint for correction (Coughlin, 1989; Newman and Fitton, 1979). The MTP joint must be considered; and if it has significant dorsiflexion, release of the dorsal capsule combined with extensor tendon lengthening should be performed in addition to the bone resection at the PIP joint.

Surgery on clawtoes and hammertoes should be done with a thigh tourniquet and not a calf tourniquet or Esmarch bandage at the ankle. The flexor muscles in the calf are preferentially squeezed by a tourniquet at this level, causing the toes to adopt a more severely clawed position. It makes satisfactory positioning of the surgically repaired toes difficult.

Proximal Hemiphalangectomy
(PIP Arthroplasty)

Technique

1. A general anesthetic is provided and a thigh tourniquet used. An elliptical incision is made over the dorsum of the PIP (Fig. 4.26), being careful not to extend it more than a one-third of the way plantarward on either side of the toe to avoid injury to the neurovascular bundles.
2. The collateral ligaments are divided along the sides of the neck of the proximal phalanx. A small bone cutter is used to make a transverse osteotomy in the neck, removing the distal 4 to 5 mm (Fig. 4.27). Use a rongeur to smooth the edges that remain.
3. Except in mild cases, an 0.062 inch K-wire is used as an internal splint to maintain alignment. It is drilled distally from the base of the middle phalanx and then in retrograde fashion into the medullary

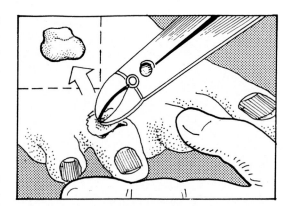

FIGURE 4.27. Proximal hemiphalangectomy (PIP arthroplasty). The head of the proximal phalanx is removed with a bone cutter through a dorsal incision.

canal of the proximal phalanx. Unless there is deformity to be corrected at the MTP joint, the K-wire should not cross that joint. The K-wire is cut just distal to the skin and a plastic cover placed over the end.
4. Regardless of whether a K-wire is used, the wound is closed with a vertical mattress stitch of 4–0 nonabsorbable suture in its center that incorporates the dorsal capsule of the PIP joint and everts the skin edges. Simple stitches are placed in the skin on either side of this central mattress stitch.

Postoperative Management. Immediate weight-bearing is allowed with a postoperative shoe, and the sutures are removed at 10 to 14 days. If a K-wire is used it is removed at 2 to 3 weeks. Athletic activities can be resumed after 4 weeks.

MTP Release

When there is dorsiflexion at the MTP joint, it must be corrected. It is generally easier to release the MTP joint and then address the PIP joint because the toe can be grasped and manuevered while working on the MTP joint.

Technique

1. A 2 cm S-shaped incision is made over the dorsum of the MTP, and the extensor tendons are identified and incised in a Z fashion.

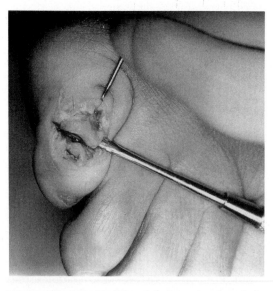

FIGURE 4.26. Proximal hemiphalangectomy of the fifth toe. The head of the proximal phalanx is exposed through a dorsal elliptical incision.

2. The dorsal MTP capsule is cut transversely and the toe plantarflexed. If it is still tight the collateral ligaments of the MTP are divided at the neck of the metatarsal. This maneuver should allow the toe to be brought into a satisfactory alignment. If there is synovitis, it is débrided with a small rongeur.
3. The PIP is then treated as described for a proximal hemiphalangectomy.
4. An 0.062 inch K-wire is inserted across the MTP joint with the toe held in a slightly plantarflexed position. The dorsal MTP capsule is left open, but the extensor tendons are repaired separately under slight tension.

Postoperative Treatment. The aftercare is the same as for a proximal hemiphalangectomy alone.

Mallet Toe

A mallet toe is characterized by an isolated, plantarflexion deformity at the DIP joint due to overpull of the long flexor tendon that inserts on the base of the distal phalanx. As with hammertoes and clawtoes, this deformity is initially flexible but can later become rigid.

Clinical Presentation

Symptoms are generally the result of corn formation on the tip of the toe or over the dorsum of the DIP joint. The deformity may be present in the second, third, or fourth toes and may affect multiple toes (Coughlin, 1995).

Nonoperative Treatment

A toe crest may support the toe and keep the tip off the insole, eliminating pain from an end corn. Moleskin or sponge pads can be placed over the corns. A more capacious toe box can prevent the shoe from rubbing against a corn on the dorsum of the DIP joint.

Operative Treatment

A flexible mallet toe can be treated with a long flexor tenotomy. Coughlin (1995) found

86% patient satisfaction with excisional arthroplasty of the DIP joint for rigid mallet toes. In cases of severe deformity, he combined the arthroplasty with flexor tenotomy through the same incision (Coughlin and Mann, 1993).

Percutaneous Long Flexor Tenotomy

Percutaneous long flexor tenotomy (Fig. 4.28) can usually be done in the office with a digital block. No tourniquet is needed.

1. A #11 scalpel is used to make a stab incision in the midline of the plantar aspect of the toe, immediately beyond the distal flexion crease. The tip of the toe is grasped and the DIP fully extended. The long flexor can then be felt against the tip of the knife blade. It is divided transversely, and the release is felt in the toe.
2. The wound is left to close secondarily, and the toe is wrapped with a pressure dressing that is removed after 3 days. Activity can be resumed after 1 week.

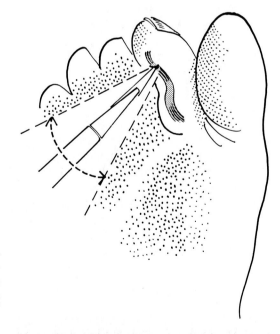

FIGURE 4.28. Percutaneous long flexor tenotomy. The long flexor is divided with a #11 scalpel at the level of the DIP joint. A back-and-forth motion is used to divide the tendon completely.

Middle Hemiphalangectomy (DIP Arthroplasty)

The middle hemiphalangectomy procedure described by Coughlin (1995) is similar to the PIP arthroplasty, performed one joint distally. Coughlin recommended removing the articular surface of the base of the distal phalanx in addition to resecting the head of the middle phalanx. The two opposing bone surfaces are then compressed, and a longitudinal K-wire is placed and left for 3 weeks. An arthrodesis is not sought with this procedure, but it occasionally occurs. The presence of arthrodesis or pseudoarthrosis has no effect on the outcome of the procedure. In instances of significant deformity, Coughlin (1995) also recommended incising the flexor tendon sheath and dividing the long flexor, done through the dorsal incision. The postoperative course is the same as for a PIP arthroplasty.

Congenital Curly Toes

Congenital curly toes is the most common lesser toe deformity in children. It usually involves the fourth and fifth toes and commonly occurs bilaterally. It is known in some cases to undergo spontaneous correction with growth (Coughlin and Mann, 1993).

Clinical Presentation

The toes are internally rotated and flexed so their lateral borders rest against the ground. The deformity is asymptomatic in most children and remains so during adulthood. When problems occur, they are due to calluses that form at the base of the nail where it rubs against the sole, or from calluses over the lateral edge of the IP joints.

Nonoperative Treatment

Taping of the toes in a corrected position with a plantar and lateral loop may hold them during athletic activities if calluses are painful. Taping does not correct the position of the toes.

Operative Treatment

Surgery is recommended in cases where taping does not relieve symptoms satisfactorily. Because deformities are flexible in children, they can be treated with flexor tenotomy of both the long and short flexor tendons (Ross and Menelaus, 1994).

Treatment is similar for adults who also have flexible deformities. If there is a fixed deformity, it is treated as a hammertoe with a proximal hemiphalangectomy (PIP arthroplasty), removing a wedge from the head of the proximal phalanx to correct the deformity.

Open Flexor Tenotomy

Technique

1. A general anesthetic is used for children, whereas in adults a digital block or ankle block is satisfactory. A transverse incision is made on the plantar aspect of the toe at the level of the PIP joint. Small retractors are placed in the wound for visualization.
2. The flexor sheath is cut transversely, and the long and short flexor tendons are divided transversely with the scalpel. If there is still a deformity, the plantar capsule of the PIP joint is also divided.
3. The skin is closed with simple stitches of 4–0 nonabsorbable suture.

Postoperative Management. A toe dressing is applied, maintaining the toe in the corrected position; and immediate weight-bearing is allowed with a postoperative shoe. The sutures are removed at 10 to 14 days and the operated toes supported with tape in the corrected position for 2 weeks. Athletic activities may then be resumed.

Overlapping or Underriding Fifth Toe

The fifth toe is unique among the lesser toes in that it has an adjacent toe on only one side. It is subject to pressures from the shoe that can force it against the fourth toe, which may lead to subluxation at the MTP joint as well as a rotational deformity that supinates the toe. The toe may finally ride up over the top of the

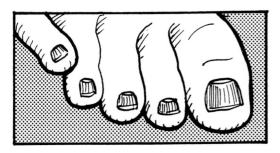

FIGURE 4.29. Overlapping fifth toe.

fourth toe (Fig. 4.29) or slip underneath it. In addition, some athletes have overlapping as a congenital deformity.

Clinical Presentation

Adult athletes may have pain caused by pressure of the toes against each other that can lead to a soft corn at the base of the web space or a hard corn distally. Some develop pain from corn formation at the lateral base of the fifth toenail if the toe has rotated enough to rub against the insole. With overlapping there may be pressure from the shoe against the top of the elevated toe.

Nonoperative Treatment

For early deformity it may be possible to tape the fifth toe down into normal alignment, using a loop over the base of the toe. A larger toebox is used to prevent lateral pressure against the toe.

With fixed deformity the toebox must accommodate the toe in its abnormal position. Sponge pads or moleskin can protect areas of corn formation. If a soft corn develops, the base of the web space should be kept open with a sponge pad more distally between the toes.

Operative Treatment

The severity of the deformity determines the surgical procedure. A mild deformity can be treated with soft tissue releases, whereas a severe deformity requires bone resection (Coughlin and Mann, 1993; Wilson, 1953). Any significant rotation of the toe qualifies as a severe deformity.

Soft Tissue Release

Technique

1. A general anesthetic is provided and a thigh tourniquet used. A Vshaped incision is made over the dorsum of the fifth MTP. The two limbs are each 1.5 cm long, and they subtend an angle of 45 degrees with the apex proximally.
2. The extensor tendon is incised in a Z fashion. The MTP capsule is cut laterally, dorsally, and as much medially as is necessary to realign the toe.
3. A 0.062 inch K-wire is inserted from the base of the proximal phalanx out through the tip of the toe. Reducing the MTP, the K-wire is drilled in retrograde fashion across the MTP joint, maintaining the toe straight. The K-wire is cut off outside the skin and covered with a plastic pin cap.
4. The medial joint capsule is then closed with 3–0 absorbable sutures, and the extensor tendon is repaired with slight tension using 2–0 absorbable suture.
5. Repositioning the toe pulls the V-shaped skin incision into a Y shape. The skin is closed with interrupted stitches of 3–0 nonabsorbable suture. A soft dressing is applied.

Postoperative Management. Immediate weight-bearing is allowed with a postoperative shoe. The skin sutures are left in place for 10 to 14 days, and the K-wire is kept in for 3 weeks. The toe should be buddy taped to the fourth toe for 3 weeks. Shoewear is advanced and athletic activity resumed after 4 weeks.

Correction

Technique. This procedure is used if there is a flexible deformity and no significant rotation of the toe.

1. A general anesthetic is provided, and a thigh tourniquet is used. A 2 cm longitudinal incision is made over the dorsum of the fifth MTP joint.
2. The extensor tendon is incised in a Z fashion. The dorsal MTP capsule is left intact, but the plantar and medial capsule are released until the toe is in a satisfactory position.

3. A 0.062 inch K-wire is drilled from the base of the proximal phalanx out through the tip of the toe. Reducing the MTP, the K-wire is drilled in retrograde fashion across the MTP joint, maintaining reduction of the toe. The K-wire is cut off outside the skin and covered with a plastic pin cap.
4. The medial joint capsule is then closed with 3–0 absorbable sutures, and the extensor tendon is repaired with slight tension using 2–0 absorbable suture.
5. A soft dressing is applied.

Postoperative Management. Immediate weight-bearing is allowed with a postoperative shoe. The skin sutures are left in place for 10 to 14 days, and the K-wire is left in for 3 weeks. The operated toe is buddy-taped to the fourth toe for 3 weeks. Shoewear is advanced and athletic activity can be resumed after 4 weeks.

Correction of Malrotation

This operative technique requires bone resection at the PIP joint. The degree of rotation is assessed, and the amount of correction required is noted. A longitudinal mark with a skin scribe is made over the dorsum of the the PIP joint, and a second parallel mark is made lateral to it, indicating the amount of correction necessary.

Technique

1. A general anesthetic is provided and a thigh tourniquet used. The procedure for a PIP arthroplasty is performed, and the distal 4 to 5 mm of the proximal phalanx head is resected.
2. The toe is rotated so the lateral mark on the distal segment is aligned with the medial mark on the proximal segment. Any tight skin is then released to allow the toe to lie in this position.
3. Proximal release is performed as for the soft tissue release about the MTP joint, as described previously.
4. A 0.062 inch K-wire is then inserted in antegrade fashion from the base of the middle phalanx, exiting the tip of the toe. It is then drilled proximally, crossing the

MTP into the metatarsal. The toe is again rotated at the PIP joint, the marks in the skin are aligned, and the wounds are closed.
5. A soft dressing is applied.

Postoperative Management. Immediate weight-bearing is started with a postoperative shoe. The skin sutures are removed at 10 to 14 days, and the K-wire is removed at 3 weeks. The toe should be buddy-taped to the fourth toe for an additional 3 weeks. Shoewear is advanced and athletic activity can be resumed after 4 weeks.

Bunionette

A bunionette is a prominence over the lateral aspect of the fifth metatarsal head that is analogous to the bunion that occurs on the medial side of the first metatarsal head. Similar to a bunion, a painful bursa can form over the prominence and cause symptoms with shoewear. Although there is often a varus position of the proximal phalanx, symptoms are usually caused by a deformity in the metatarsal. Bunionettes often occur in the same foot with hallux valgus and bunion; this combination is termed a splay foot.

Clinical Presentation

Symptoms from a bunionette are caused by the shoe rubbing against the lateral prominence. A painful bursa may develop that increases the size of the prominence, leading to increased pain. A plantar callus may also form in conjunction with the lateral prominence.

Radiography

Three recognized patterns are associated with bunionettes (Coughlin, 1991). There may be a large prominence of the fifth metatarsal head (type I), or the metatarsal may have a lateral bow that makes a normally shaped head protrude laterally (type II). The head may also protrude owing to an increased divergence between the fourth and fifth metatarsals (type III).

Nonoperative Treatment

Accommodative shoes are the mainstay of initial treatment for bunionettes. As with bunions, relief of pressure on the prominence usually eliminates the pain. However, shoes that have a wide toebox often do not provide enough support to allow athletic activities. Leather shoes can be stretched over the prominence, or cutouts and balloon patches can be applied.

Operative Treatment

If the weight-bearing AP radiograph shows that the deformity is caused by a lateral prominence of the metatarsal head (type I), a simple exostectomy may be sufficient (Kitaoka, 1992). If the fifth metatarsal is bowed (type II) or there is an increased intermetatarsal 4–5 angle (type III), an osteotomy should be performed. Osteotomies have been described for the distal, middle, and proximal metatarsals to treat bunionettes (Coughlin, 1991; Diebold, 1991; Diebold and Bejjani, 1987; Kitaoka and Holiday,1992; Kitaoka et al., 1991; Kitaoka and Leventer,1989; Moran and Claridge, 1994). Proximal osteotomies have the potential for poor bone healing if they damage the nutrient artery (Smith et al., 1992). Oblique midshaft osteotomies yield good results but are unstable and require internal fixation (Coughlin, 1991). In fact, the deformity can be satisfactorily treated with a distal fifth metatarsal chevron-type osteotomy (Kitaoka et al., 1991; Moran and Claridge, 1994).

Simple Exostectomy

Technique

1. A general anesthetic or ankle block is administered, and a tourniquet is used. A 3 cm straight lateral incision is made over the bunionette, and dorsal and plantar flaps are developed.
2. The lateral joint capsule is split longitudinally in line with the skin incision, incising superior to the tendinous insertion of the abductor digiti quinti minimi. The capsule is elevated dorsally and plantarward to expose the metatarsal head.

3. A small oscillating saw is used to cut the lateral prominence, directed from distal to proximal. The cut should be made in line with the lateral shaft of the metatarsal. In cases where there is a prominent lateral condyle of the proximal phalangeal base, it is trimmed. The bone edges are smoothed with a rongeur.
4. The lateral capsule edges are then trimmed so the closure is taut. The capsule is sutured with interrupted 3–0 absorbable suture. The skin is closed with a running stitch of 3–0 nonabsorbable suture. A soft dressing is applied.

Postoperative Management. Immediate weight-bearing is allowed in a postoperative shoe. The skin sutures are removed at 10 to 14 days, and shoewear is advanced. Return to athletic activities is allowed 3 weeks after surgery.

Fifth Metatarsal Chevron Osteotomy

Technique

1. A general anesthetic or ankle block is administered, and an appropriate tourniquet is used. A 3 cm straight lateral incision is made over the bunionette (Fig. 4.30), and dorsal and plantar flaps are developed.
2. The lateral joint capsule is split longitudinally in line with the skin incision, incising superior to the tendinous insertion of the abductor digiti quinti minimi. The capsule is elevated dorsally and plantarward to expose the metatarsal head.
3. A small oscillating saw is used to cut the lateral prominence, directed from distal to proximal. The cut should be made in line with the lateral shaft of the metatarsal.
4. The center of the metatarsal head is identified, and a small K-wire is used to drill a transverse hole in its center. This hole marks the apex of the chevron cut.
5. A V-shaped cut is made in the head of the metatarsal with the small oscillating saw such that the two limbs of the chevron form an angle of 60 degrees. The head fragment that remains is small, and care must be taken to avoid cutting into it with the saw blade.

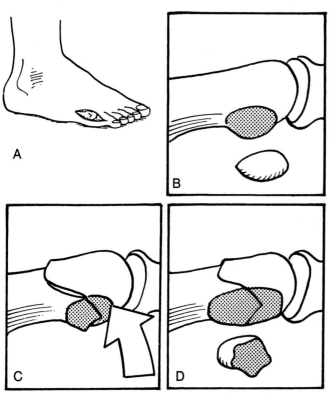

FIGURE 4.30. Chevron correction of a bunionette. (A) Incision is placed laterally over the fifth metatarsal head. (B) Lateral prominence of the metatarsal head is excised with an oscillating saw. (C) After making a V cut with the apex in the center of the metatarsal head, the head segment is displaced medially. (D) Exposed prominence of the distal metatarsal shaft segment is removed with the saw, cutting parallel to the lateral border of the head segment.

6. The head fragment is translated medially 3 to 4 mm and impacted onto the metatarsal shaft segment with axial pressure applied distal to proximal along the toe. The head should translate medially only and should not be allowed to displace dorsally or plantarward.
7. The oscillating saw blade is then directed in a distal to proximal direction using the lateral surface of the head fragment as a guide. The exposed lateral segment of the metatarsal shaft is cut, leaving a smooth lateral border of the distal fifth metatarsal.
8. The edges of the lateral capsule are then trimmed so the closure is taut. The capsule is closed with 3–0 absorbable sutures. The osteotomy and capsule closure provide adequate stability, so fixation with a K-wire is not usually required. The skin is closed with a running stitch of 3–0 nonabsorbable suture. A soft dressing is applied.

Postoperative Management. Immediate weight-bearing is allowed with a postoperative shoe. The sutures are removed at 10 to 14 days, and a postoperative shoe is worn for 3 weeks before shoewear is advanced. Athletic activities should be avoided until 6 weeks after surgery.

Lesser Toe Fractures and Dislocations

Fractures

Most lesser toe fractures occur when the individuals are barefoot and the toe is stubbed (axially loaded) against a stationary object. Athletic shoes generally protect the toes from this type of injury. Objects dropping on the shod toe, however, can cause phalangeal fractures. The proximal phalanx is that most commonly fractured; and when stubbing is the cause, the fifth toe, which is unprotected laterally, is typically injured (De-Lee, 1993; Elleby and Marciko, 1985).

Clinical Presentation

These fractures are painful and associated with a traumatic event that can be easily described. The toe is swollen, tender, and usually ecchymotic. Gross malalignment is uncommon. A crush injury or violent force directed against the toe may cause an open fracture.

Radiography

Routine radiographs confirm the diagnosis; and AP, lateral, and oblique views are obtained to ensure that an associated dislocation is not missed (Fugate et al., 1991). The usual fracture descriptions (closed versus open, nondisplaced versus displaced, angulated, intraarticular) apply to toe fractures, as do the principles of fracture management.

Nonoperative Treatment

Most lesser toe fractures can be satisfactorily treated by buddy taping the fractured toe to the adjacent toe. The uninjured acts as a splint, and the relative immobilization protects the toe, promoting healing and decreasing pain. A postoperative stiff-soled, or regular shoe can be utilized, depending on the athlete's level of pain. Pain typically is present for 2 to 3 weeks, but swelling can continue for 2 to 3 months. Advancement of shoewear and return to athletic activities is based on the level of pain.

Operative Treatment

Open fractures of the toes require the same treatment as other open fractures. A povidone–iodine soaked sterile dressing is applied on the field. Antibiotics and, if indicated, tetanus toxoid are administered in the emergency room. Culture specimens are obtained in the operating room.

Thorough irrigation and débridement comprise the first step for treating this injury in the operating room. The wound must be left open to close secondarily. If the alignment is satisfactory, soft dressings are applied until the skin has healed, followed by buddy-taping. These measures are sufficient to maintain the position of the fracture. Percutaneous K-wires are used if there is gross comminution or marked instability of the fracture.

Closed fractures that are significantly angulated or are associated with dislocation of a joint benefit from closed reduction, followed by maintenance of the position with buddy taping or percutaneous K-wire fixation. Open reduction is rarely indicated for toe fractures.

Dislocations

Dislocation is an uncommon injury that usually involves the fifth toe (DeLee, 1993; Jahss, 1981b). An abduction force applied to the toe is the usual cause. MTP dislocation is more likely to occur than IP dislocation (Fugate et al., 1994; Weinstein and Insler, 1994). The distal joint (IP) is stable to abduction stress, whereas the proximal joint (MTP) is mobile. Therefore an abduction stress on the toe has a longer moment arm to act on the MTP joint, in contrast to the IP, and can exert a greater force.

Clinical Presentation

There is usually swelling that may be accompanied by ecchymosis. The toe appears deviated, although significant swelling may mask it. Attempted motion, both passive and active, are painful. Palpation may reveal abnormal alignment of the joint along with tenderness, which is typical.

Radiography

Anteroposterior and lateral radiographs of the toes are necessary to reveal the deformity and to exclude associated fracture.

Treatment

Nonoperative Treatment. A closed reduction should be attempted, and if the treatment is rendered soon after the injury, it will probably be successful. The position is then held by buddy-taping to an adjacent toe. The swelling may make manipulation of the toe and maintenance of the reduction difficult. If the toe can be reduced but then the reduction is lost, longitudinal K-wire fixation of the toe for 2 weeks should be used. If the toe cannot be reduced closed, open reduction and K-wire fixation should be performed.

Technique

1. A digital block with 1% lidocaine is performed at the level of the MTP joint to reduce the risk of additional swelling at the site of the IP dislocation. It can be done in the office or clinic.
2. The proximal phalanx is stabilized, and traction is applied through the tip of the toe. The distal toe is then translated to effect the reduction. Radiographs are obtained to ensure that the position is satisfactory.
3. Buddy-taping is applied and the toe supported in this manner for 2 weeks. A regular shoe may be worn as soon as it fits. Athletic activities can be resumed immediately if the toe is securely taped.

Operative Treatment. If the reduction slips, K-wire fixation should be performed. It must be done in an operating room.

1. After administering an appropriate anesthetic, the proximal phalanx is stabilized and traction applied through the tip of the toe. The distal toe is then translated to effect the reduction.
2. After reducing the dislocation, a 0.062 inch K-wire is drilled from the tip of the toe through the intramedullary spaces of the phalanges, without entering the MTP joint.
3. Radiographs are obtained to assess the reduction and implant position. A postoperative shoe is worn for 2 weeks, at which time the pin is removed (in the office) and shoewear and activities are advanced.

Open Reduction

1. Appropriate anesthesia is provided, and a tourniquet is used. A transverse incision is made over the dorsum of the dislocated IP joint, dividing the extensor apparatus and dorsal capsule of the joint.
2. With longitudinal traction the toe should be reducible. Any soft tissue blocking reduction is divided.
3. A 0.062 inch K-wire is drilled from the tip of the toe through the intramedullary spaces of the phalanges, extending to but not crossing into the MTP joint. Radiographs are obtained to assess the reduction and implant position.

4. The skin is closed with interrupted 4–0 nonabsorbable sutures. A postoperative shoe is worn for 2 weeks, at which time the sutures and pin are removed and shoewear and activities are advanced.

Acute Metatarsal Fracture

Acute metatarsal fractures are caused by a specific traumatic episode. The mechanism of injury can usually be clearly described. The shaft of the metatarsal fractures as the result of a direct blow, from dropping an object on the foot or having it stepped on. There may be a violent twisting or wrenching action on the forefoot with the hindfoot fixed. Conversely, the forefoot may be fixed while the hindfoot is twisted. Pathologic fractures can occur through bone abnormalities caused by tumor or infection.

If the fracture causes the metatarsal head to heal in a displaced, plantar position, a prominence results, which can lead to the development of a callus or intractable plantar keratosis. Conversely, a dorsally displaced metatarsal head can lead to a dorsal prominence, which is likely to rub against the top of the shoe. Dorsal displacement may also cause a transfer metatarsalgia under the adjacent metatarsal heads by altering of the normal pattern of weight-bearing. Lateral translation of the metatarsal head is generally well tolerated, although neuritic symptoms may develop from pressure on the intermetatarsal nerve traveling through a narrowed interspace.

Clinical Presentation

The athlete may note a pop with an associated sharp pain that prevents weight-bearing. The physical examination may show swelling and ecchymosis either dorsally or plantarward. There is point tenderness over the fracture. Rapid swelling precludes the ability to determine the degree and direction of fracture displacement.

Radiography

Standard AP, lateral, and oblique radiographs of the foot clearly show the fracture and allow determination of comminution, displacement, and angulation. It is especially important to evaluate the position of the head of the fractured metatarsal on the lateral radiograph.

Nonoperative Treatment

Most metatarsal shaft fractures can be treated by nonoperative methods. Fractures that are not displaced or only minimally displaced can be treated by protection in a stiff-soled or postoperative shoe, allowing immediate weight-bearing. Symptoms usually resolve by 3 to 4 weeks. Crutches are useful for the first few days during which progressive weight-bearing is allowed based on pain. A short-leg walking cast or walking orthosis provides more support and is used for 1 to 2 weeks if pain is significant. Prolonged use of a cast is not indicated for minimally displaced fractures owing to the osteopenia, stiffness, and muscle atrophy that can result. An orthosis may be used for a longer period but should be regularly removed for motion exercises several times each day.

Displaced metatarsal fractures in which the metatarsal head has not translated dorsally or plantarward can be treated in a similar fashion. Displacement of the metatarsal head up to 4 mm can be safely treated without an attempt at reduction. Athletic activities should be avoided until 6 weeks after most acute metatarsal fractures.

Operative Treatment

Operative treatment is reserved for the metatarsal shaft fracture that has significant displacement of the head, has severe dorsal angulation that is tenting the skin, is open, or occurs with other metatarsal fractures with displacement (DeLee, 1993). Single or multiple closed fractures can usually be treated with closed reduction and casting, although irreducible ones require open reduction and fixation with K-wires or small fragment plates. Open fractures must be irrigated, reduced, and internally fixed. Fractures as the result of crush injuries may have an associated compartment syndrome, which must be evaluated and treated concomitantly (Myerson, 1988, 1991, 1993).

Closed Reduction

1. A general anesthetic is used to provide muscle relaxation, thereby easing the reduction. Each toe is wrapped with adhesive tape and then placed in Chinese finger traps.
2. The foot is suspended from the finger traps for 5 to 10 minutes, allowing longitudinal traction to effect a satisfactory reduction. Intraoperative radiographs are obtained to verify the position.
3. Manual reduction of the fracture is attempted if suspension alone does not reduce the fracture. If manipulation is unsuccessful, open reduction is undertaken (see below).
4. After reduction, a short-leg cast is applied and weight-bearing allowed as tolerated. The foot is protected in a cast for 4 weeks. The initial cast may be changed after 7 to 10 days if it is loose owing to reduced swelling. A postoperative shoe is then worn for 2 weeks, after which activities can be advanced.

Open Reduction and Fixation

Technique

1. Appropriate anesthesia is given, and a tourniquet is used. A 5 to 6 cm longitudinal incision is made on the dorsum of the foot over the fractured metatarsal. If two metatarsals are fractured, the incision is made between them; if three, the incision is made over the central one. If there is concern about compartment syndrome, incisions are made over the second and fourth metatarsals, through which the compartments can also be released.
2. Superficial nerves and extensor tendons are protected, and the dorsal veins are divided only as necessary. The fractures are exposed with minimal elevation of the interosseous muscles.
3. Reduction is performed, and 0.062 inch K-wires are used for fixation. An intraoperative radiograph is obtained to verify the reduction and the K-wire position.
4. If fixation is adequate, the wires are cut off outside the skin and the wound closed in layers.

4. Alternatively, fixation can be performed with small fragment lag screws with or without a dorsal neutralization plate.

5. When treating open metatarsal fractures with reduction and fixation the skin must be left open, and delayed primary closure or coverage with a split-thickness skin graft is performed at 5 to 7 days.

Postoperative Management. After closure, a short-leg cast is applied. The skin sutures are removed at 10 to 14 days, and a new cast is applied. If K-wires have been used for fixation, they are removed at 6 weeks and weight-bearing is allowed in a postoperative shoe. Shoewear can be advanced as tolerated. Athletic activities should be delayed until 8 weeks after surgery.

If internal fixation with screws has been performed, a walking orthosis is applied after the skin sutures have been removed. Motion exercises can be started immediately. A regular shoe is worn after 6 weeks, and athletic activities are begun at 8 weeks after surgery.

Forefoot Compartment Syndrome

When trauma to the foot causes multiple metatarsal fractures, particularly as the result of a crushing injury, compartment syndrome must be excluded. The forefoot musculature is divided into four compartments bordered by the metatarsals and fascial planes. Intracompartmental pressure can rise considerably after trauma due to bleeding and fluid extravasation. This situation, in turn, can result in vascular impairment, and if untreated it can lead to myonecrosis, scarring, and fibrosis. The sequelae of this chain of events includes chronic pain and loss of forefoot function.

Direct vascular injury may lead to compartment syndrome. This has been described in a volleyball player who suffered an inversion ankle injury that caused a pseudoneurysm of the dorsalis pedis artery and subsequent compartment syndrome (Kym and Worsing, 1990). Exertional compartment syndromes of the feet are rare but have been reported, both acute and chronic. In one case it followed a vigorous aerobic exercise session (Middleton et al., 1995). In another, it appeared gradually over a period of six months in a ballet dancer (Lokiec et al., 1991). A high degree of suspicion is necessary to correctly diagnose this problem.

Anatomy

The forefoot is divided into four compartments (Fig. 4.31) by the metatarsal and inter-

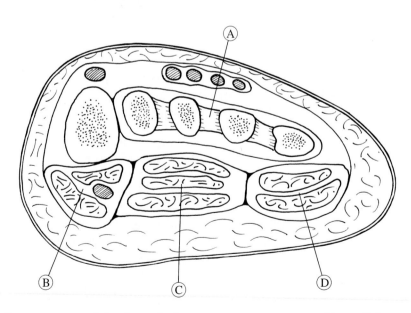

FIGURE 4.31. Compartments of the foot. A, Interosseous compartment; B, medial compartment; C, central compartment; D, lateral compartment.

connecting fascial planes (Meyerson, 1988). The interosseous compartment is in the dorsum of the foot. It is defined by the lateral aspect of the first metatarsal and medial aspect of the fifth metatarsal and is surrounded by the interosseous fascia. It contains the second through fourth metatarsals and the seven interosseous muscles. The medial compartment is bordered above by the undersurface of the first metatarsal, medially and inferiorly by the plantar aponeurosis, and laterally by an intermuscular septum. It contains the abductor hallucis and flexor hallucis brevis muscles. The central compartment is bordered above by the interosseous compartment, medially and laterally by intermuscular septae, and inferiorly by the plantar aponeurosis. It contains the abductor hallucis, quadratus plantae, lumbrical, and flexor digitorum brevis muscles. The lateral compartment is bordered by the fifth metatarsal dorsally, the plantar aponeurosis inferiorly and laterally, and an intermuscular septum medially. It contains the flexor, abductor, and opponens muscles for the fifth toe.

Clinical Presentation

The diagnosis of compartment syndrome requires a high index of suspicion. Tense swelling in the forefoot is typical, usually as the result of crush injuries. Pain on passive stretching of the toes or dysesthesias in the toes are not reliable signs of compartment syndrome in the foot.

The diagnosis is confirmed by wick catheter measurements of intracompartmental pressures, which should be obtained for all four compartments. Indications for compartment release are pressures above 30 mm Hg or pressures 30 mm Hg below the diastolic blood pressure (DeLee, 1993; Meyerson, 1991, 1993).

Measurement of Forefoot Compartment Pressures

See Myerson (1991) for more detailed information.

1. Kits are available that provide slit catheters and hand-held monitors for measuring compartment pressure. Alternatively, a slit catheter can be attached to a transducer and the pressure obtained with an arterial line manometer setup. The slit catheter apparatus is first zeroed and then inserted sequentially into the four compartments of the foot.
2. The interosseous compartment is first entered by placing an 18 gauge 1.5 inch needle between the second and third metatarsals dorsally, passing into the muscle. The tip should not be in contact with the bone. The catheter is then placed through the needle and the pressure measured.
3. The needle is advanced down into the muscle of the central compartment, the catheter reinserted. and the pressure recorded.
4. The medial compartment pressure is measured by placing the needle just inferior to the first metatarsal into the flexor hallucis brevis muscle belly.
5. The lateral compartment pressure is measured by placing the needle inferior to the fifth metatarsal into the abductor digiti quinti muscle.

Forefoot Compartment Release

See Myerson (1988, 1993) for more detailed information.

1. When compartment syndrome has been diagnosed, it is treated using two incisions on the dorsum of the foot. Longitudinal incisions of 6 cm each are made over the dorsum of the second and fourth metatarsals.
2. Blunt dissection between each of the metatarsals reveals the underlying interosseous fascia, which is sharply divided longitudinally. Further dissection under the first and fifth metatarsals is necessary to ensure that the medial and lateral compartments have been adequately released.
3. The metatarsal fractures are then treated with reduction and fixation as indicated. The incisions should be left open, covered with sterile dressings, and a short-leg posterior splint applied. A delayed primary closure or coverage by split-thickness skin grafting is performed at 5 to 7 days.

References

Axe MJ, Ray RL: Orthotic treatment of sesamoid pain. Am J Sports Med 16:411–416, 1988

Barbari SG, Brevig K: Correction of clawtoes by the Girdlestone-Taylor flexor-extensor transfer procedure. Foot Ankle 5:67–73, 1984

Baxter DE: Treatment of bunion deformity in the athlete. Orthop Clin North Am 25:33–39, 1994

Braddock G: Experimental epiphyseal injury and Freiberg's disease. Bone Joint Surg Br 41:154–159, 1959

Clanton TO, Butler JE, Eggert A: Injuries to the metatarsophalangeal joints in athletes. Foot Ankle 7:162–176, 1986

Coker TP, Arnold JA, Weber DL: Traumatic lesions of the metatarsophalangeal joint in the great toe in athletes. Am J Sports Med 6:326–334, 1978

Coughlin MJ: Juvenile bunions In: Mann RA, Coughlin MJ (eds): Surgery of the Foot and Ankle, pp 467–543, St. Louis, Mosby, 1993a

Couglin MJ: Operative repair of the mallet toe deformity. Foot Ankle 16:109–116, 1995

Coughlin MJ: Second metatarsophalangeal joint instability in the athlete. Foot Ankle 14:309–319, 1993b

Coughlin MJ: Subluxation and dislocation of the second metatarsophalangeal joint. Orthop Clin North Am 20:535–551, 1989

Coughlin MJ: Treatment of bunionette deformity with longitudinal diaphyseal osteotomy with distal soft tissue repair. Foot Ankle 11:195–203, 1991

Coughlin MJ, Mann RA: Lesser toe deformities. In Mann RA, Coughlin MJ (eds): Surgery of the Foot and Ankle pp 341–412. St. Louis, Mosby, 1993

DeLee JC: Fractures and dislocations of the foot. In: Mann RA, Coughlin MJ (eds): Surgery of the Foot and Ankle, pp 1465–1703. St. Louis, Mosby,1993

Diebold PF: Basal osteotomy of the fifth metatarsal for thebunionette. Foot Ankle 12:74–79,1991

Diebold PF, Bejjani FJ: Basal osteotomy of the fifth metatarsal with intermetatarsal pinning: a new approach to tailor's bunion. Foot Ankle 8:40–45, 1987

Dietzen CJ: Great toe sesamoid injuries in the athlete. Orthop Rev 19:966–972, 1990

Douglas G, Rang, M: The role of trauma in the pathogenesis of the osteochondroses. Clin Orthop 158:28–34,1981

Einarsdottir H, Troell S, Wykman A: Hallux valgus in ballet dancers: a myth? Foot Ankle 16:92–94, 1995

Elleby DH, Marcinko DE: Digital fractures and dislocations: diagnosis and treatment. Clin Podiatry 2:233–245, 1985

Fugate DS, Thomson JD, Christensen KP: An irreducible fracture-dislocation of the lesser toe: a case report. Foot Ankle 11:317–318, 1991

Gauthier G, Elbaz R: Freiberg's infraction: a subchondral bone fatigue fracture; a new surgical treatment. Clin Orthop 142:93–95,1979

Gould N: Hallux rigidus: cheilectomy or implant? Foot Ankle 1:315–320, 1981

Hattrup SJ, Johnson KA: Chevron osteotomy: analysis of factors in patients' dissatisfaction. Foot Ankle 5:327–332, 1985

Hawkins BJ, Haddad RJ: Hallux rigidus. Clin Sports Med 7:37–49, 1988

Helal B, Gibb P: Freiberg's disease: A suggested pattern of management. Foot Ankle 8:94–102,1987

Holmes GB, Timmerman L: A quantitative assessment of the effects of metatarsal pads on plantar pressures. Foot Ankle 11:141–145, 1990

Howse J: Disorders of the great toe in dancers. Clin Sports Med 2:499–505, 1983

Irvin CM, Witt, CS, Zielsdorf LM: Post-traumatic osteochondritis of the lateral sesamoid in active adolescents. J Foot Surg 24:219–221, 1985

Jahss MH: Chronic and recurrent dislocations of the fifth toe. Foot Ankle 1:275–278, 1981a

Jahss MH: Stubbing injuries to the hallux. Foot Ankle 1:327–332, 1981b

Jahss MJ: Traumatic dislocations of the first metatarsophalangeal joint. Foot Ankle 1:15–21, 1980

Johnston RB, Smith J, Daniels T: The plantar plate of the lesser toes: an anatomical study in human cadavers. Foot Ankle 15:276–282, 1994

Jones, KJ, Feiwell LA, Freedman EL, Cracchiolo A: The effect of chevron osteotomy with lateral capsular release on the blood supply to the first metatarsal head. J Bone Joint Surg Am 77:197–204, 1995

Katcherian DA: Treatment of Freiberg's disease. Orthop Clin North Am 25:69–81, 994

Kinnard P, Lirette R: Dorsiflexion osteotomy in Freiberg's disease. Foot Ankle 9:226–231, 1989

Kitaoka HB, Franco MG, Weaver AL, Ilstrup DM: Simple bunionectomy with medial capsulorrhaphy. Foot Ankle 12:86–91, 1991

Kitaoka HB, Holiday AD, Campbell DC: Distal chevron metatarsal osteotomy for bunionette. Foot Ankle 12:80–85, 1991

Kitaoka HB, Holiday, AD: Lateral condylar resection for bunionette. Clin Orthop 278:183–192, 1992

Kitaoka HB, Leventen EO: Medial displacement metatarsal osteotomy for treatment of painful bunionette. Clin Orthop 243:172–179, 1989

Kliman ME, Gross E, Pritzker KPH, Greyson ND: Osteochondritis of the hallux sesamoid bones. Foot Ankle 3:220–223, 1983

Kym MR, Worsing RA: Compartment syndrome in the foot after an inversion injury to the ankle. Bone Joint Surg Am 72:138–139, 1990

Lavery LA, Harkless LB: The interpositional athroplasty procedure in treatment of degenerative arthritis of the second metatarsophalangeal joint. J Foot Surg 31:590–594, 1992

Leventen EO: Sesamoid disorders and treatment: an update. Clin Orthop 269:236–240, 1991

Lewis AG, DeLee JC: Type I complex dislocation of the first metatarsophalangeal joint, reduction through a dorsal approach. J Bone Joint Surg Am 66:1120–1123, 1984

Lillich JS, Baxter DE: Bunionectomies and related surgery in the elite female middle-distance and marathon runner. Am J Sports Med 14:491–493, 1986

Lokiec F, Siev-ner I, Pritsch M: Chronic compartment syndrome of both feet. J Bone Joint Surg Br 75:178–179, 1991

Lutter, LD: Running athlete in office pratice. Foot Ankle 3:53–59, 1982

Mann RA, Clanton TO: Hallux rigidus: treatment by cheilectomy. J Bone Joint Surg Am 70:400–406, 1988

Mann RA, Coughlin MJ: Adult hallux valgus. In: Mann RA, Coughlin MJ (eds): Surgery of the Foot and Ankle, pp 167–296. St Louis, Mosby, 1993a

Mann RA, Coughlin MJ: Keratotic disorders of the plantar skin. In: Mann RA, Coughlin MJ (eds): Surgery of the Foot and Ankle, pp 413–465. St. Louis, Mosby, 1993b

McBride ID, Wyss UP, Cooke TD: First metatarsophalangeal joint reaction forces during high-heel gait. Foot Ankle 11:282–288, 1991

McBryde AM: Sesamoid foot problems in the athlete. Clin Sports Med 7:51–60, 1988

McBryde AM, Anderson RB: Sesamoid foot problems in the athlete. Clin Sports Med 7:51–60, 1988

McDermott EP: Basketball injuries of the foot and ankle. Clin Sports Med 12:373–393, 1993

McMaster M: The pathogenesis of hallux rigidus. J Bone Joint Surg Br 60:82–87, 1978

Middleton DK, Johnson JE, Davies JF: Exertional compartment syndrome of bilateral feet: a case report. Foot Ankle 16:95–96, 1995

Moran MM, Claridge RJ: Chevon osteotomy for bunionette. Foot Ankle 15:684–688, 1994

Myerson, MS: Experimental decompression of the fascial compartments of the foot—the basis for fasciotomy in acute compartment syndromes. Foot Ankle 8:308–314, 1988

Myerson MS: Management of compartment syndromes for the foot. Clin Orthop 271:239–248, 1991

Myerson MS: Soft-tissue trauma—acute and chronic management. In: Mann RA, Coughlin MJ (eds): Surgery of the Foot and Ankle, pp 1367–1410. St. Louis, Mosby, 1993

Myerson MS, Shereff MJ: The pathological anatomy of claw and hammer toes. J Bone Joint Surg 71:45–49, 1989

Newman RJ, Fitton JM: An evaluation of operative procedures in the treatment of hammer toe. Acta Orthop Scand 50:709–712, 1979

Rau FD, Manoli A: Traumatic boutonniere deformity as a cause of actue hammer toe: a case report. Foot Ankle 11:231–232, 1991

Richardson, EG: Injuries to the hallucal sesamoids in the athlete. Foot Ankle 7:229–244, 1987

Rodeo SA, Warren, RF, O'Brien SJ, et al: Diastasis of bipartite sesamoids of the first metatarsophalangeal joint. Foot Ankle 14:425–434, 1993

Ross ERS, Menelaus MB: Open flexor tenotomy for hammer toes and curly toes in children. J Bone Joint Surg Br 66:770–771, 1984

Sammarco GJ: Forefoot conditions in dancers: part I. Foot ankle 3:85–92, 1982

Sammarco GJ: Turf toe. AAOS Instruct Course Lect 42:207–212, 1993

Sammaro GJ, Miller EH: Forefoot conditions in dancers: part II. Foot Ankle 3:93–98, 1982

Sarafian SK: Anatomy of the foot and ankle: topographical, functional and descriptive. Philadelphia, Lippincott, 1983

Sarrafian SK, Topouzian LK: Anatomy and physiology of the extensor apparatus of the toes. J Bone Joint Surg Am 51:669–679, 1969

Scranton PE: Pathological anatomic variations in the sesamoids. Foot Ankle 1:321–326, 1981

Scranton PE, Rutkowski, R: Anatomic variations in the first ray. Part II] Disorders of the sesamoids. Clin Orthop 151:256–264, 1980

Smillie I: Freiberg's infraction (Koehler's second disease). J Bone Joint Surg Br 39:580, 1957

Smith JW, Arnoczky SP, Hersh A: The intraosseous blood supply of the fifth metatarsal: implications for proximal fracture healing. Foot Ankle 13:143–152, 1992

Smith RW, Reischl SF: Metatarsophalangeal joint synovitis in athletes. Clin Sports Med 7:75–88, 1988

Sobel M, Hashimoto J, Arnoczky SP, Bohne

WHO: The microvasculature of the sesamoid complex: its clinical significance. Foot Ankle 13:59–363, 1992

Teitz CC, Harrington RM, Wiley H: Pressure on the foot in pointe shoes. FootAnkle 5:216–221, 1985

Tewes DP, Fischer DA, Fritts HM, Guanche, CA: MRI findings of acute turf toe: a case report and review of anatomy. Clin Orthop 304:200–203,1994

Thompson F, Hamilton WG: Problems of the second metatarsophalangeal joint.Orthopaedics 10:83–89,1987

Thompson FM, Mann RA: Arthritides. In Mann RA, Coughlin MJ (eds): Surgery of the Foot and Ankle, pp 615–671. St. Louis, Mosby, 1993

Van Hal ME, Keene JS, Clancy WG: Stress fractures of the great toe sesamoids. Am J Sports Med 10:122–128,1982

Vittetoe DA, Saltzman CL, Krieg JC, Brown TD: Validity and reliability of the first distal metatarsal articular angle. Foot Ankle 15:541–547, 1994

Weinstein RN, Insler HP: Irreducible proximal interphalangeal dislocation of the fourth toe: a case report. Foot Ankle 15:627–629,1994

Wiley J, Thurston P: Freiberg's disease. J Bone Joint Surg Br 63:459, 1981

Wilson JN: V-Y correction for varus deformity of the fifth toe. Br J Surg 41:133–135, 1953

Wolfe J, Goodhart C: Irreduible dislocation of the great toe following a sports injury. Am J Sports Med 17:695–696, 1989

Zimmer TJ, Johnson KA, Klassen RA: Treatment of hallux valgus in adolescents by the chevron osteotomy. Foot Ankle 9:190–193, 1989

5
Tendon Disorders

Achilles Tendonitis and Partial Tears

Achilles tendonitis is a common overuse problem found in a variety of athletes. Its incidence has been noted to be as high as 18% in a group of runners (Krissoff and Ferris, 1979). Any athlete who is involved in repetitive impact loading from running or jumping is at risk for developing Achilles tendonitis (Clain and Baxter, 1992).

Tendonitis describes a spectrum of injuries to the Achilles tendon. Paratendinitis is inflammation of the tendon sheath. Tendinosis indicates degeneration within the substance of the tendon itself. Intratendinous calcification occasionally occurs in the calcaneal insertion. These various pathologic conditions may occur separately or in combination, but all can be considered Achilles tendonitis (Cain and Baxter, 1992; Clancy et al., 1976; Kvist et al., 1987; Nelen et al., 1989; Scoli, 1994; Smart et al., 1980).

History

Most athletes describe the gradual onset of pain just above the tendo Achilles insertion, sometimes associated with a recent change in training conditions or activities. Runners who increase their mileage or intensity of workouts, change shoes, or work out on a new training surface are at risk for developing tendonitis. Poor warm-up and warm-

down can also lead to irritation and tendonitis. The athlete should be questioned about these factors to determine causation and to identify ways for preventing recurrence.

Physical Examination

Acutely, the physical examination reveals tenderness to palpation over the tendon that may be either pinpoint or diffuse. As the problem becomes chronic, the tenderness becomes more diffuse and may be associated with a fusiform swelling palpable in the tendon (Scoli, 1994). The entire heel should be examined with care to localize additional foci of tenderness.

Partial tear of the tendon is usually associated with an acute episode of pain and weakness in the calf. The finding of significant swelling or thickening or a palpable defect in the tendon, however, should alert the examiner to the possibility of a partial or even complete rupture (Fig. 5.1).

Radiography

Routine radiographs, particularly a lateral view of the heel, can demonstrate calcification within the tendon. The contour of the calcaneus is assessed to determine if a prominent superior tuberosity is contributing to tendon irritation (Haglund syndrome).

Magnetic resonance imaging (MRI) can be helpful when evaluating defects or swelling to determine if there has been a partial or complete tear, or if scarring or fluid is present

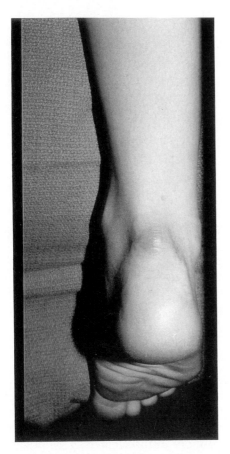

FIGURE 5.1. Large nodule on the Achilles tendon of a volleyball player.

and activity is impaired, a walking orthosis or cast for 2 to 4 weeks to completely rest the tendon may be needed (Smart et al., 1980).

A short course of a nonsteroidal antiinflammatory drug (NSAID) for 1 to 2 weeks can dramatically reduce symptoms (Cain and Baxter, 1992). Use of a heel lift of 0.25 to 0.50 inch reduces stress on the tendon. Women can be advised to wear high-heel shoes during the day when not training.

A program of ice massage and interferential electrical stimulation can be instituted. As symptoms begin to resolve, gentle stretching exercises are helpful for restoring tendon length and are preparatory for the strengthening programs necessary before returning to activity. Calf strengthening begins with double-toe and then single toe raises. In the athlete with chronic tendonitis stretching can be started immediately. Warm-up and warmdown stretching must be adopted by the athlete when activity is resumed.

Steroids are not injected into the Achilles tendon or about its insertion. The physician who is intimately aware of the anatomy may be comfortable about injecting steroid exactly into the retrocalcaneal bursa. However, it is still possible for some to extravasate about the tendon. The result may be necrosis of the tendon and rupture (Fig. 5.2) (Kleinman and Gross, 1983).

Operative Treatment

Surgery is indicated for the treatment of calcific tendonitis and chronic painful tendinosis unresponsive to nonoperative measures. Athletes with chronic swelling and thickening of the tendon that does not respond to nonoperative measures should undergo an MRI examination. Thickening of the paratenon, which indicates paratenonitis can be treated by excision of the paratenon and lysis of adhesions (Kvist et al., 1987). If there is evidence of a cyst, scarring, or chronic tendinitis within the substance of the tendon that does not involve the entire width of the tendon (Fig. 5.3), the abnormal tissue can be excised and the normal tendon repaired (Clancy et al., 1986). If there is full-thickness disruption of the tendon over a short length,

in the substance of the tendon. If surgical treatment of an intrasubstance tear (tendinosis) is under consideration, MRI can demonstrate the extent of scarring (Marcus et al., 1989).

Ultrasonography is another modality that can identify scarring and edema within the tendon. It has the disadvantage, however, that it is operator-dependent (Maffulli et al., 1987).

Nonoperative Treatment

As with other overuse injuries, the most important factor in treating Achilles tendonitis is rest. Mild cases may respond to an interval reduction in duration and intensity of activity. More significant involvement usually requires complete cessation of the activity for 1 to 2 weeks. If symptoms persist

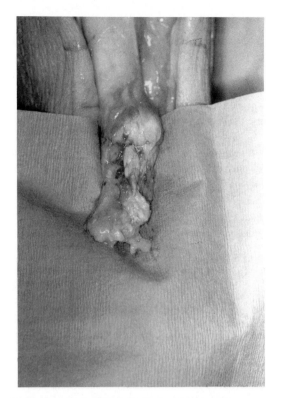

FIGURE 5.2. Complete rupture of the tendon after a steroid injection by another physician.

it may be possible to excise the segment and perform a primary repair, similar to repairing an acute rupture (Nelen et al., 1989; Skeoch, 1981). If more than 2 cm must be excised, however, the repair requires a reconstruction procedure using a turn-down flap or aug-

mentation with a tendon transfer (Cain and Baxter, 1992; Clancy et al., 1976; Nelen et al., 1989; Wapner et al., 1993).

Excision of Scarred Achilles Tendon Tissue and Paratenon

Technique

1. A general anesthetic is given and a thigh tourniquet applied. The procedure is performed with the patient in the prone position. A longitudinal incision is made along the medial side of the Achilles tendon extending 6 to 10 cm, centered over the distal tendon.
2. The paratenon is split longitudinally over the area identified by radiography or MRI as the site of the pathology. Any thickened paratenon is excised, and adhesions are débrided sharply with a scalpel.
3. If there is intrasubstance pathology, the tendon is also split in line with its fibers until the abnormal tissue is identified. It is then excised until only normal tissue remains. Any calcified tissue can be identified by its feel, whereas the scar is recognized by its uniform white appearance, different from the striated normal tendon. If a cyst is present, it is also excised.
4. The defect in the normal tendon is then repaired with a nonstrangulating running stitch of 0 absorbable suture. The paratenon is reapproximated using 2–0 absorbable su-

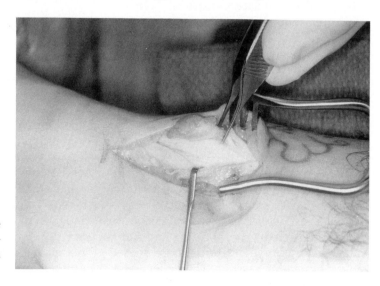

FIGURE 5.3. Partial rupture of the Achilles tendon. Note the segment of abnormal tendon with a cyst posteriorly.

ture and the skin closed with a subcuticular suture or interrupted mattress sutures.

Postoperative Management. A short-leg splint or cast is applied and the patient kept non-weight-bearing for 10 to 14 days. The skin sutures are removed, and weight-bearing is allowed in a removable walking orthosis. The orthosis is worn for 4 weeks, during which time it is removed regularly several times a day for range of motion exercises. At this point, formal therapy with modalities and light resistive exercises can be started. Most athletes are able to return to practice by 8 to 10 weeks.

Excision of a Segment of Achilles Tendon (< 2 cm)

Technique

1. A general anesthetic is used and a thigh tourniquet placed. The procedure is performed with the patient in the prone position. A longitudinal incision is made along the medial side of the Achilles tendon, extending 10 to 12 cm.
2. The paratenon is split longitudinally over the area of the defect identified on MRI. The abnormality is identified and excised. The defect remaining must be *less* than 2 cm in length.
3. The tendon is repaired as for an acute tear. Sutures of no. 2 nonabsorbable material are woven in Bunnell-like manner along the medial and lateral sides of both the proximal and distal ends of the tendon. With the foot in no more than 20 degrees of equinus, the sutures are securely tied, holding the ends apposed. The repair is augmented with multiple stitches of 0 absorbable suture. The paratenon is repaired with 2–0 absorbable suture and the skin closed.

Postoperative Management. A short-leg equinus cast is applied and the patient maintained non-weight-bearing for 10 to 14 days. The skin sutures are removed; and a removable orthosis, which blocks dorsiflexion, is applied. Protected weight-bearing and early, gentle range of motion exercises are started and continued for 6 weeks. Thereafter, reha-

bilitation follows the same protocol as for complete ruptures (see Achilles Tendon Rupture, below).

Achilles Tendon Rupture

Rupture of the Achilles tendon is a significant and potentially career-ending injury. Stiffness, loss of push-off power, and rerupture are complications. Although some individuals have had preceding symptoms from tendonitis or a partial tear, most cases are spontaneous. In athletes, basketball and racquet sports account for most of these injuries.

Pathogenesis and Injury

Naturally occurring degenerative changes and diminished blood supply to the tendon just proximal to its insertion combine to cause potential weakness in the Achilles tendon (Carr and Norris, 1989; Kannus and Jozsa, 1991). When the tendon is overloaded (usually by an excessive dorsiflexion force) while the gastrocnemius-soleus muscle unit is contracting (as during push-off), rupture can occur.

Clinical Presentation

Characteristic of rupture is an audible pop, which occurs during push-off. Immediate, severe pain may or may not occur. Some patients note only weakness with push-off and an inability to run, whereas others are unable to walk without a limp. Eventually, swelling and ecchymosis are usually present and may extend to the medial and lateral borders of the foot. Numbness in the sural nerve distribution is not an uncommon complaint.

Physical examination is performed with the patient prone. On inspection there is usually swelling and ecchymosis unless the patient is seen immediately. Palpation along the Achilles tendon is painful. A gap may be appreciated, or hematoma may fill the sheath, simulating an intact tendon. Although active plantar flexion is diminished after rupture, it is rarely absent. Unless the Thompson squeeze test is performed, the examiner may be misled and the diagnosis missed (Thompson and Doherty, 1962). The test is performed by squeezing the calf immediately distal to its maximum girth to elicit plantarflexion of the ankle. If the Achilles tendon is ruptured, the ankle does not plantarflex, and the test is considered positive. An alternative test for integrity of the Achilles uses a sphygmomanometer placed around the calf and inflated to 100 mm Hg (Copeland, 1990). As the ankle and foot are then passively moved by the examiner from plantarflexion to dorsiflexion, the pressure increases approximately 40 mm Hg when the tendon is intact.

Radiography and MRI

Routinely, anteroposterior (AP) and lateral radiographic views of the ankle are obtained. They usually indicate soft tissue swelling only, but occasionally calcification within the tendon or at its insertion are noted. MRI is not normally performed for clinically evident complete rupture, although it may be of benefit in patients being considered for nonoperative treatment by demonstrating apposition of the torn tendon ends when the ankle and foot are plantarflexed.

Nonoperative Treatment

A torn Achilles tendon can heal with immobilization of the foot and ankle in equinus (Nistorm 1981). The major disadvantages of nonoperative treatment include loss of power (decreased plantarflexion strength), increased risk of rerupture, and an overall decreased rate of return to the prior level of sport activity (Cetti et al., 1993).

For the patient who declines surgical intervention and for athletes over age 40, we have used nonoperative treatment with good results. To approximate the torn tendon ends, the ankle is plantarflexed to 10 degrees of maximum and then immobilized in a well padded short-leg cast for 4 weeks. A new cast with the ankle immobilized in plantarflexion of only 10 degrees is then used for another 4 weeks. At 8 weeks the patient's shoes are fitted with a 0.5-inch heel lift for another 4 week period. Use of a stationary bicycle is permitted at the end of cast immobilization.

Unrestricted range of motion exercises are permitted at 8 weeks, but plantarflexion resistive exercises are not initiated until 12 weeks after the injury. Single-leg toe raises are started at 16 weeks. Running on a treadmill is allowed at this point, and transition to running and jumping usually occurs by 5 to 6 months. Sport specific drills lead to return to sports, usually between 8 to 9 months.

Operative Treatment

The major advantages of operative repair include a higher rate of return to activity, increased plantarflexion strength, and decreased calf atrophy (Cetti, 1993; Inglis et al., 1976). Disadvantages of operative treatment include anesthetic complications, infection, sensory nerve injury, and wound healing problems (hematoma, skin necrosis, and adhesions) (Cetti et al., 1993). In general, surgical repair of the Achilles tendon is the recommended treatment. Although percutaneous repair is effective (Ma and Griffith, 1977), open repair appears to have a lower incidence of rerupture and is used in most athletes (Bradley and Tibone, 1990).

Acute Repair of Achilles Rupture

Technique

1. Repair is undertaken with the patient prone after an epidural or general anesthetic has been administered.
2. A longitudinal incision is made along the posteromedial border of the Achilles tendon, centered over the defect. This incision offsets the scar from the posterior aspect of the distal leg, which may improve gliding, and allows access to the plantaris tendon (it is if needed to reinforce the repair). This approach also limits the chance of injuring the sural nerve, which is located posterolaterally. The skin and subcutaneous tissue are sharply incised to the paratenon, which is distended with hematoma. Avoid creating flaps, which can lead to skin necrosis and scar adhesion.
3. Incise the paratenon carefully so it can be repaired later. Hematoma is removed by gentle débridement and irrigation. Identify

the torn ends of the Achilles tendon, which typically resemble mop ends (Fig. 5.3). Do not débride tendon fibers, but an overtly degenerative and cystic focus through which rupture has occurred can be débrided.

4. Plantarflex the ankle and foot to reapproximate the tendon ends. An end-to-end repair is then performed using two or more #2 nonabsorbable sutures, inserted in a whip-stitch configuration (Fig. 5.4). The sutures are tied while the knee is flexed to 90 degrees and the foot and ankle are placed in 10 degrees of plantarflexion. The ankle and foot should then be able to be brought to neutral with palpable tension in the repaired tendon but without gaping at the repair site.

5. Once the core repair has been performed, use a running 0 absorbable suture to coapt the superficial fibers around the entire tendon circumference.

6. Repair the paratenon with a 2–0 absorbable running stitch. If the paratenon cannot be reapproximated, detach the plantaris tendon proximally in the calf, leaving it attached to the calcaneus. Using fine he-

mostats, spread the tendon out into a broad sheet, which is then applied circumferentially around the repair site (Lynn, 1966).

7. Close the subcutaneous tissue with inverted, interrupted stitches, using a 3–0 absorbable suture. The skin is closed with a subcuticular stitch, using a 3–0 absorbable suture. A well padded, short-leg posterior splint is applied, maintaining the ankle and foot in 10 degrees of plantarflexion. The patient can usually be discharged from the hosptial within 24 hours of surgery. Non-weight-bearing ambulation and elevation of the operated leg as much as possible is advised.

Postoperative Management. At 1 week inspect the wound. Usually, healing of the skin has been sufficient to allow bathing. With a satisfactory repair, early, limited ankle motion is possible (Mandelbaum et al., 1995), which is beneficial for improving tendon healing as well as decreasing potential stiffness. Using a dorsal block splint, active motion is allowed from neutral to as much plantarflexion as tolerated. Dorsiflexion is strictly prevented.

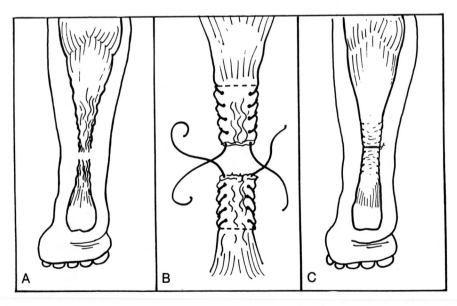

FIGURE 5.4. Repair of Achilles tendon rupture. (A) Ruptured Achilles tendon. (B) Whipstitch woven along the sides of the tendon with the ends of the suture in the gap between the tendon ends. (C) Sutures are tied, bringing the ends of the tendon together.

A removable, fiberglass dorsal shell or a commercial orthosis, which prevent dorsiflexion motion, are used. The dorsal block splint or orthosis is removed three times daily for exercise periods of 15 minutes each. If the patient is thought to be unreliable or the repair questionable, however, use a short-leg cast with the ankle in 5 to 10 degrees of equinus for 6 weeks.

Protected weight-bearing is used for a total of 4 to 6 weeks. Weight-bearing using a 0.5-inch heel lift is then started. Full, unrestricted active range of motion exercise, including dorsiflexion, is allowed at 6 weeks. Swimming and stationary cycling are begun at 8 weeks. The heel lift is discontinued at 10 weeks. Resistive dorsiflexion exercises are started at 10 weeks with light tubing. At 12 weeks double toe raises against only body weight are initiated and progressed to single-leg raises as strength develops. Rope jumping is a useful exercise for strengthening the calf muscles at this point. Running is usually possible by 4 to 5 months. Return to basketball, volleyball, or other sports that require repetitive explosive jumping is not allowed until 9 months after surgery.

Chronic Rupture of the Achilles Tendon

Neglected ruptures, partial ruptures that subsequently progress to full-thickness tears, and ruptures associated with steroid injections (Mahler and Fritscy, 1992) typically are associated with intervening scar tissue. The latter, after excision, result in the inability to perform end-to-end repair. To bridge the defect, peroneus brevis (White and Kraynick, 1959), fascia lata (Bosworth, 1956), turn-down of a portion of the proximal Achilles tendon, V-Y gastrocplasty (Abraham and Pankovich, 1975), and transfer of the flexor digitorum longus to the calcaneus (Mann et al., 1991) have been used. Turn-down of a strip of the proximal Achilles tendon (Fig. 5.5) has been successful in our experience.

Technique

1. With the patient prone make a posteromedial longitudinal incision approximately the length of the tendon from the calcaneus to the musculotendinous junction. Incise the subcutaneous tissues without creating flaps, exposing the sheath and tendon.
2. Excise scar and granulation tissue (Fig. 5.5B). If the gap is too great to achieve apposition of the tendon ends primarily, a proximal turn-down flap is needed (Fig. 5.5C).
3. If the distal tendon insertion into the calcaneus is insufficient for suture, the turn-down flap must be brought through a transverse drill hole in the calcaneus (Fig. 5.5D). Use a 4.5 mm drill bit and enlarge the tunnel as needed.
4. Pass the graft, place the ankle in 20 degrees of plantarflexion, and after pulling the graft tight suture it to itself (Fig. 5.5E). Proximally, place a stitch, using #2 nonabsorbable suture, at the apex of the flap to prevent potential distal extension of the defect, which can cause loss of adequate tension in the reconstruction.
5. Usually the sheath cannot be closed. The plantaris tendon, which is left attached distally, is teased apart into a broad, thin sheet and incorporated around the reconstructed Achilles tendon.
6. The subcutaneous tissues and skin are closed in layers. A short-leg, medio-lateral U splint with a posterior foot plate, maintaining the ankle and foot at 20 degrees of plantarflexion, is applied.

Postoperative Management

The sutures are removed at 1 week. A short-leg weight-bearing cast with the ankle at 20 degrees of plantarflexion is worn for five additional weeks. A 0.5-inch heel lift is then used for another 4 weeks, but the patient is allowed to perform active range of motion exercises between plantarflexion and neutral. At 8 weeks, passive motion and soft tissue mobilization are begun to regain as much dorsiflexion as possible. Bicycling and treadmill walking are started. Plantarflexion resistive exercises are delayed until 3 months. A permanent loss of power is typical, although most athletes can run and jump, usually at a lower level than before injury. Return to sports requires a minimum of 12 months.

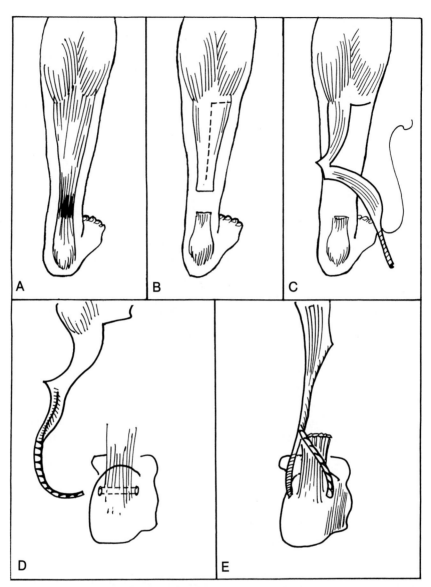

FIGURE 5.5. Reconstruction of Achilles tendon with a turn-down flap. (A) Achilles tendon with pathologic segment (dark area). (B) Excision of abnormal tissue, leaving normal ends of the tendon proximally and distally. The flap to be turned is outlined (dotted line). (C) After turning down the flap the distal end is trimmed and tubularized. (D) End of the flap is passed through a transverse drill-hole in the calcaneus. (E) Tendon is sutured back onto itself.

Peroneal Tendon

Dislocation

Dislocation of the peroneal tendon occurs not infrequently when skiing or playing basketball. Often the dislocation is not diagnosed acutely. Peroneal tendon injuries should be considered in the differential diagnosis of a lateral ankle ligament injury. Of added importance is the occasional occurrence of longitudinal tears of the peroneal tendons in conjunction with tendon dislocation.

Anatomy

The peroneal tendons are routed from the distal leg to the foot within a groove of varying depth in the posterior aspect of the inferior fibula. In this groove, the tendons are constrained by the superior peroneal retinaculum, which attaches to the periosteum of the distal fibula.

Pathomechanics

Two mechanisms of injury are encountered. Forced dorsiflexion of the foot resisted by strong peroneal contraction or inversion of the plantarflexed foot and ankle can result in either frank rupture of the superior peroneal retinaculum or stripping of the periosteal attachments of the retinaculum, thereby causing a redundant sheath which allows the tendons to subluxate or dislocate anterior to the distal fibula.

Clinical Presentation

Acute Dislocation

With acute dislocation the patient usually notes pain localized to the lateral and posterior ankle. A pop may have been felt or heard, and a subsequent click with walking is noted. If the injury is examined early, swelling may be retromalleolar but later becomes generalized over the lateral side of the ankle. Direct tenderness can be noted along the retromalleolar course of the peroneal tendons. It is infrequent that subluxation or dislocation of the tendons is observed with active eversion and dorsiflexion. The examiner must be aware that lateral ankle injuries and peroneal tendon dislocation can occur concomitantly.

Chronic Dislocation

With chronic dislocation most patients complain of a feeling of ankle instability with pivoting and twisting rather than dislocation of the tendons. Pain and clicking may be present. The diagnosis is established by passive subluxation or dislocation of the peroneal tendons by the examiner or its observation on active eversion and dorsiflexion of the foot and ankle by the patient (Fig. 5.6).

Radiography and MRI

Routine radiographs can exclude ankle fractures; however, only on an internal oblique view of the ankle can possible avulsion from the peroneal groove be demonstrated. MRI is beneficial for identifying associated tears of the peroneal tendons.

Treatment

Acute injuries may respond to 6 weeks of immobilization in a short-leg walking cast. Incorporating a lateral horseshoe pad constructed of felt or similar material is useful for

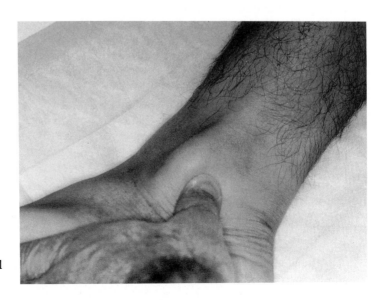

FIGURE 5.6. Dislocatable peroneal tendons.

maintaining the peroneal tendons posteriorly. This step is followed by range of motion exercises and peroneal isometric and resistive strengthening exercises. Early surgery may be elected because of the predictable success of the operation and the minimal increase in time to return to sports compared to closed treatment. If so, the stabilization procedure described below is utilized.

Chronic peroneal dislocation most often requires surgical treatment in athletes. A number of surgical procedures have been used succesfully to stabilize dislocation of the peroneal tendons. Essentially, these procedures either reconstruct the peroneal retinaculum or deepen the peroneal groove by a bone block osteotomy, sliding graft, or osteoperiosteal flap. We have found local reconstruction of the peroneal retinaculum to be a reliable method of stabilization.

Peroneal Tendon Stabilization

Technique. The technique is illustrated in Figure 5.7.

1. Under tourniquet control and with a bump placed underneath the ipsilateral hip, start an incision 2 cm distal to the lateral malleolus tip over the peroneal tendons. Extend this 3 cm proximal to the tip, staying immediately posterior to the fibula to avoid the sural nerve.
2. Incise the peroneal sheath anteriorly, leaving a small cuff attached to the fibula. Inspect the peroneal tendons for pathologic changes. Repair significant longitudinal tears (usually involving the peroneus longus) using 2–0 absorbable mattress sutures.
3. Mobilize the lateral flap of the peroneal sheath and place two horizontal mattress sutures (2–0 nonabsorbable suture) in it such that the free ends of the sutures exit the external surface of the lateral flap.
4. At the midpoint of the peroneal groove drill four holes, 1.5 mm in diameter, that exit on the anterior surface of the fibula. Pass the sutures into the drill holes.
5. With the ankle in neutral, tie the sutures over their bony bridges. Check that ankle motion is full. If not, the repair is too tight,

and the sutures must be retied more loosely.
6. Close the skin with interrupted simple mattress sutures (3–0 nylon) and apply a well padded U-splint or posterior splint to the leg, ankle, and foot.

Postoperative Management. Remove the sutures at 10 to 14 days. At that time a short-leg weight-bearing cast is applied for a total of 6 weeks of immobilization. Then commence therapy with emphasis on range-of-motion of both the ankle and subtalar joints and strengthening of the dorsiflexor and peroneal tendons especially. Return to activity averages 3 months from surgery. No special taping or bracing is required.

Tendonitis and Tears

Peroneus Longus

The peroneus longus tendon is infrequently the site of athletic injury, but it must be considered in cases of lateral midfoot and hindfoot pain. Injuries to the peroneus longus tendon include acute rupture with or without os peroneum fracture, stenosing tenosynovitis secondary to a healed os peroneum fracture, and attritional intra-substance tears in the tendon (Fig. 5.8). These injuries have been grouped together under the term painful os peroneum syndrome by Sobel et al. (1994).

Anatomy

Beyond the lateral malleolus, the peroneus longus travels to the level of the cuboid. There an oval accessory bone, the os peroneum, lies within its substance. The os peroneum is always present, though it is ossified and radiologically visible in only 5% to 20% of the population (Sarrafian, 1983; Sobel et al., 1994). The os peroneum is tethered to the calcaneus, cuboid, fifth metatarsal base, and plantar fascia with soft tissue attachments (Peterson and Stinson, 1992; Sarrafian, 1983; Sobel et al., 1994).

Distal to this point the tendon passes under the cuboid in a tunnel formed by a groove in the cuboid and covered by the long

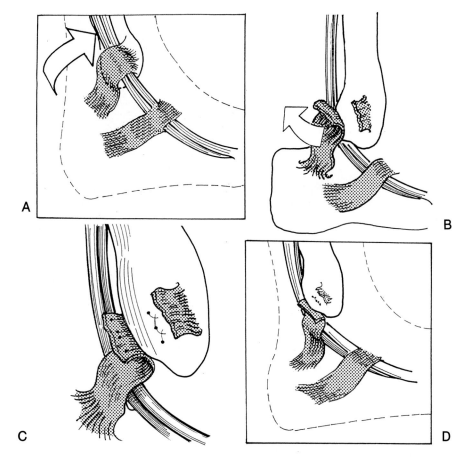

FIGURE 5.7. Repair of dislocating peroneal tendons. (A) Peroneal tendons have slipped anteriorly over the lateral malleolus with an incompetent superior peroneal retinaculum. (B) Division of the superior peroneal retinaculum, leaving a cuff attached to the fibula. The tendons have been replaced in their groove behind the malleolus. (C) Sutures are passed through the retinaculum and drill holes in the posterior fibula. (D) Superior peroneal retinaculum is fixed to the posterior fibula by tying the sutures.

plantar ligament; it then traverses under the foot to attach to the plantar base of the first metatarsal and medial cuneiform. The muscle functions to evert and pronate the foot and plantarflex the first metatarsal (Sammarco, 1994).

Clinical Presentation

Symptoms of peroneal tendon pathology occur both acutely and chronically. When acute rupture occurs, it follows a traumatic event with an inversion and plantarflexion mechanism (Peterson and Stinson, 1992). Tenderness and swelling are noted along the course of the peroneus longus inferior to the lateral malleolus, though eversion of the foot and plantarflexion of the first metatarsal may be intact (Kilkelly and McHale, 1994).

Chronic symptoms are not infrequently associated with lateral ankle instability or peroneal tendon dislocation and are due to attritional tears of the tendon and healing fractures or diastasis of the os peroneum (Sobel et al., 1994). The lateral hindfoot pain can be associated with swelling over the tendon below the malleolus and pain on single-toe raises. Tenderness and crepitus may be present along the course of the tendon as well.

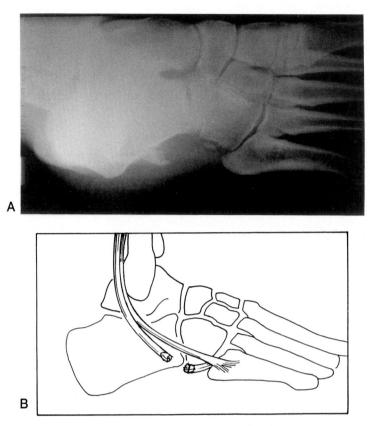

Figure 5.8. Peroneus longus rupture through the os peroneum. The os peroneum is fractured, and the proximal piece has retracted. (A) Radiograph. (B) Illustration.

Radiography

The oblique radiograph of the foot can be useful for excluding a fracture of the os peroneum, when ossified. MRI can identify intrasubstance tears of the tendon as well as complete disruption (Kilkelly and McHale, 1984; Mink et al., 1991; Sammarco, 1994).

Nonoperative Treatment

Tendonitis of the peroneus longus is readily treated with a period of rest and oral anti-inflammatory medication. Use of a short-leg walking cast for 3 to 4 weeks may prove helpful in difficult cases. A longitudinal arch support with medial posting to prevent pronation can be used for a short period when activities are resumed (Sammarco, 1994). These measures are less successful in treating intrasubstance tears.

Operative Treatment

Surgery is often necessary if there is significant pain and weakness associated with a tendon tear or rupture or with os peroneum fracture. Intrasubstance tears are treated by excision of the defect and primary repair, and ruptures can be treated by primary repair if the injury is acute or tenodesis to the peroneus brevis if it is chronic (Kilkelly and McHale, 1994; Sammarco, 1994; Sobel et al., 1994; Thompson and Patterson, 1989). Fracture of the os peroneum without tendon disruption is treated by excising the accessory bone (Peterson and Stinson, 1992).

Technique

1. A general anesthetic is administered and a thigh tourniquet applied. A curvilinear incision is made from the tip of the lateral

malleolus to the base of the fifth metatarsal. The sural nerve is identified and protected.

2. The peroneal sheath is entered, and the peroneus brevis and peroneus longus tendons are inspected.

3. If there are attritional tears in the substance of the tendon, the degenerated tissue is excised and the defect closed with a running stitch of 2–0 absorbable suture.

4. If an acute rupture of the peroneus longus is present, the ends are freshened and primarily repaired using a Bunnell-like stitch of #1 nonabsorbable suture.

5. If the rupture is chronic, regardless of whether the os peroneum is fractured, the degenerated ends of the tendon and the os peroneum are excised. A side-to-side anastomosis of the proximal and distal ends of the peroneus longus to the peroneus brevis tendon is performed with multiple stitches of #1 nonabsorbable suture.

6. If the tendon is intact but the os peroneum has fractured, the fractured fragments are shelled out from the tendon and the defect repaired with 2–0 absorbable sutures.

7. In all cases, the peroneal sheath and retinaculum are repaired with 2–0 absorbable sutures, the skin closed, and a posterior splint applied.

Postoperative Management. No weight-bearing is permitted for 10 to 14 days, at which time the skin sutures are removed. A short-leg cast is applied with the foot in slight eversion for an additional 4 weeks. A short-leg walking orthosis is then worn for 4 to 6 weeks with removal several times a day for range-of-motion exercises and therapeutic modalities. Peroneal resistive exercises are not permitted until 8 to 10 weeks. Athletic activities can be resumed as early as 3 months after surgery.

Peroneus Brevis Tendon

Unlike dislocation, tendinitis/partial rupture of the peroneus brevis tendon is infrequently encountered and only recently has been described as a clinical entity. It is typically the consequence of an inversion injury of the ankle, and its symptoms resemble those associated with a lateral ankle sprain.

The peroneus brevis muscle pronates and everts the foot. Underneath the tip of the fibula its tendon undergoes a shift in direction. This change, together with potential abrasion from a bony or cartilaginous ridge along the undersurface of the malleolus, limited vascularity of the tendon underneath the malleolus, and a prominent calcaneofibular ligament, has been implicated in the development of peroneus brevis tendinitis and tears. (Meyer, 1924; Sammarco, 1994; Sammarco and DeRaimondo, 1989; Scheller et al., 1980; Sobel et al., 1994; Trevino and Baumhauer, 1992).

Tendinitis is associated with swelling within the tendon sheath. Partial tears of the tendon are usually longitudinal fissures that may be single or multiple and are found in the area of the tip of the lateral malleolus (Fig. 5.9) (Sammarco, 1994; Trevino and Baumhauer, 1992). These tears have been noted to affect the anterior or middle portion of the tendon (Jones, 1993).

Clinical Presentation

Tendinitis/partial rupture may occur acutely following an inversion injury, or it may present with chronic symptoms. In the latter instance, there may have been a remote inversion injury that caused the process to develop subclinically. When it occurs acutely, the athlete notes lateral ankle pain and

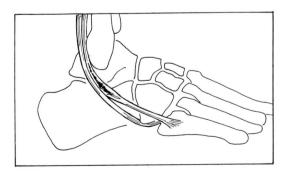

FIGURE 5.9. Longitudinal tear in the peroneus brevis inferior to the lateral malleolus.

swelling similar to that of an inversion sprain; chronic injury is more likely to cause weakness or giving-way when cutting and jumping than pain, which is referred to the lateral ankle. With an acute injury the examination reveals swelling in the tendon sheath, and both acute and chronic injuries present with tenderness along the peroneal tendons underneath the lateral malleolus. Manual muscle testing of foot eversion can be painful and weak. Associated lateral ankle instability, demonstrated clinically or radiographically, has been described (Sammarco and DeRaimondo, 1989). Despite these findings, the diagnosis may prove elusive.

Radiography

Routine radiographs are normal. Peroneal tenography may show a partial tear in the tendon, but this procedure is invasive (Trevino and Baumhauer, 1992). MRI can demonstrate swelling within the tendon sheath with either tendinitis or a partial tear (Sammarco, 1994). With a tear, an increased signal within the tendon and alteration of normal morphology can be noted (Mink et al., 1981).

Nonoperative Treatment

Tendinitis is treated with activity restriction, oral NSAIDs, and occasionally a period of non-weight-bearing immobilization. If symptoms do not resolve, surgical synovectomy is offered to the patient.

Operative Treatment

Symptoms that are not responsive to non-operative measures should alert the physician to the possibility of a partial tear in the tendon. Tears generally require surgical treatment (Jones, 1993). At the time of surgery the tendon is assessed and treatment individualized. If the tendon is normal, synovectomy alone is performed. If there is only a small slip of tendon torn, it is removed. A larger, centrally located tear can be treated with excision of the edges and primary repair. If the entire tendon is involved, particularly if it is significantly frayed, the abnormal tendon

segment is excised, and the normal tendon above and below are tenodesed to the peroneus longus tendon. Any associated instability of the ankle should be addressed at the same time, with delayed repair or reconstruction of the lateral ankle ligaments.

Technique

1. An appropriate general or regional anesthetic is administered. The patient is positioned supine with a bump placed under the ipsilateral hip. A thigh tourniquet is used.
2. A 7 to 10 cm incision is made along the course of the peroneus brevis tendon beginning 1 to 2 cm proximal to the tip of the malleolus. The peroneal tendon sheath is split longitudinally in its center, extending from distal to the lateral malleolus, allowing the superior peroneal retinaculum to be advanced into the malleolus if any redundancy of the retinaculum exists.
3. The peroneus brevis and longus tendons are then inspected.
4. If the tendons appear normal, a synovectomy is performed to remove the synovial lining of the sheath.
5. If there is a tear that has a small slip separated from the bulk of the tendon, this slip is simply excised.
6. If the tear is larger and more centrally located in the tendon, the edges are excised on both sides with a scalpel. The defect is then closed with a running stitch of 2–0 absorbable suture.
7. If the entire tendon is involved and frayed, the pathologic segment is excised. The proximal and distal stumps are sutured side-to-side to the peroneus longus tendon with interrupted stitches using a #1 nonabsorbable suture.
8. The peroneal sheath is then closed with a running stitch of 0 absorbable suture. The wound is closed and a posterior splint applied.

Postoperative Management

Crutches are used for 10 to 14 days, at which point the splint and skin sutures are removed. If a synovectomy alone has been performed or if a small slip of tendon was excised, the athlete wears a removable walking orthosis for 3 to 4 weeks, performing range of motion exercises and receiving therapeutic modalities. If a tear has been repaired or a tenodesis performed, a short-leg walking cast is applied and worn for 4 weeks. Return to activity follows restoration of motion and maximal gains in strength and proprioception.

Posterior Tibialis Tendon

Injury to the posterior tibialis tendon, common in middle-aged individuals, frequently leads to a flatfoot deformity (Funk et al., 1986; Johnson and Strom, 1989). Although older athletes are particularly susceptible, injury can also occur in younger athletes. Types of injuries include the rare acute rupture, insertional tendonitis, and tenosynovitis that may lead to partial or complete rupture and ultimately a flatfoot deformity (Fig. 5.10). (Conti, 1994; Funk et al., 1986; Johnson and Strom, 1989; Monto et al., 1991; Woods and Leach, 1991).

Anatomy and Function

The posterior tibialis muscle lies in the deep posterior compartment of the leg, and its tendon passes directly behind the medial malleolus in a synovial sheath to attach to the medial pole of the navicular. Small slips of the tendon also attach to the plantar aspect of the three cuneiforms, the cuboid, and the medial three metatarsal bases. A zone of hypovascularity exists in the tendon in the area just distal to the medial malleolus (Frey et al., 1990).

The posterior tibialis muscle is an important dynamic stabilizer of the longitudinal arch (Conti, 1994). It acts during the foot-flat interval of the stance phase of gait with eccentric contraction, followed by concentric contraction through the toe-off interval (Mann, 1993). When posterior tibialis function is lost, collapse of the medial longitu-

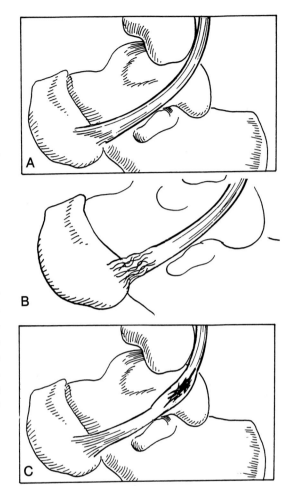

FIGURE 5.10. Tibialis posterior tendon injury. (A) Normal course of the posterior tibialis tendon as it travels under the medial malleolus to insert along the navicular. (B) Insertional tendonitis of the posterior tibialis. (C) Partial rupture with a longitudinal fissure and swelling just inferior to the malleolus.

dinal arch results with a flatfoot deformity and inability to support the body with toe raise.

Pathomechanics

The etiology of tendon rupture is unknown. One theory is that mechanical irritation against the undersurface of the medial malleolus is the cause. Alternatively, as the tendon changes direction underneath the

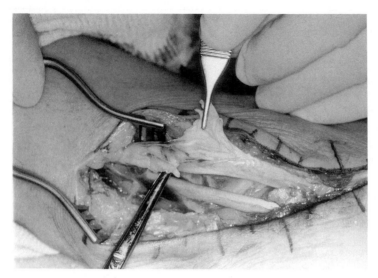

FIGURE 5.11. Partial rupture of the posterior tibialis tendon. The tendon is frayed and substantially torn. The flexor digitorum longus tendon is seen running behind it, already harvested for a tendon reconstruction procedure.

malleolus it may be chronically stressed, eventually leading to rupture. Finally, the existence of the hypovascular area underneath the malleolus may contribute to tendon disruption (Fig. 5.11).

Clinical Presentation

The usual presentation of posterior tibialis tendon pathology is a gradual onset of medial hindfoot or arch pain. It may be present for months with only mild to moderate functional limitation. Examination of the foot during this time reveals tenderness and slight swelling along the course of the tendon from the medial malleolus to the navicular. There may be discomfort with single-leg toe raises on the affected side, corresponding to tenosynovitis in the tendon sheath (Johnson and Strom, 1989; Trevino and Baumhauer, 1992).

This stage is followed by an abrupt or rapid decrease in function and increase in pain. There is still tenderness and swelling and now an inability to perform single-leg toe raises. At this point there has been a tear in the tendon, either a partial intrasubstance tear or a complete rupture.

The final phase occurs over the ensuing several months as the plantar ligaments are gradually stretched during weight-bearing with a nonfunctional posterior tibialis tendon. It causes loss of the longitudinal arch with prominence of the head of the talus in the medial hindfoot and abduction of the forefoot.

Radiography

Routine radiographs of the foot and ankle are usually obtained to exclude other causes of hindfoot pain. Tenosynovitis and tendon rupture cannot be diagnosed on plain radiographs. MRI is an excellent test for evaluating posterior tibialis tendon pathology. Tenosynovitis demonstrates fluid within the tendon sheath without disruption of the tendon itself. Tendon tears are classified as one of three types based on MRI findings (Mink et al., 1991). Type I has longitudinal splits within the tendon and appears swollen or hypertrophic. Type II also has longitudinal splits, but the tendon appears thin or atrophic. This phase is probably a prerupture stage. Type III demonstrates complete rupture of the tendon.

Nonoperative Treatment

Tenosynovitis is treated by a combination of rest and antiinflammatory medication. The rest is provided with activity limitation or cessation or cast immobilization for 3 to 4 weeks. Steroid injections are contraindicated, as they have been implicated in rupture of the posterior tibialis tendon (Trevino et al.,

1981). If there is incomplete relief after cast immobilization, synovectomy and inspection of the tendon are indicated.

If longitudinal tears have occurred in the tendon but it remains in continuity, a course of cast immobilization can be attempted. It is unlikely to be successful, however, and surgery is necessary to restore function. Similarly, a frank rupture, regardless of the presence of hindfoot deformity, is associated with significant functional loss that cannot be restored without surgery. Accommodation with a brace allows pain relief and some restoration of function but not enough to allow further participation in athletic activities.

Operative Treatment

Surgery of posterior tibialis tendon pathology begins with open synovectomy of the tendon sheath. At that time the tendon is inspected; and if a small intrasubstance tear is found, it is excised and the tendon primarily repaired. Large repairs or frank ruptures require reconstruction with transfer of the flexor digitorum longus tendon. If the arch has collapsed, a soft tissue procedure alone is inadequate for restoring hindfoot function, and hindfoot fusion is necessary.

Synovectomy of Posterior Tibialis Tendon Sheath

Technique

1. A general anesthetic is administered and a thigh tourniquet applied. A curvilinear incision is made over the course of the tendon posterior to the malleolus, beginning proximally 3 to 4 cm and extending distally immediately beyond the navicular.
2. The tendon sheath is identified and split longitudinally from the navicular to the proximal extent of the wound with scissors. With synovitis there is typically bulging fluid, and the synovium is thickened and inflamed. The synovial lining of the sheath is removed with scissors.
3. The tendon is inspected for any defects that can be repaired if small. A tear with a

rim of normal tendon tissue is excised with a #15 scalpel. If the remaining tendon is more than one-half its normal diameter, direct repair is possible. The defect is closed with a running 2–0 absorbable suture. If the remaining tendon is smaller than one-half its original diameter it should be reconstructed with a flexor digitorum longus tendon transfer.
4. At this point the sheath is closed with a running 2–0 absorbable suture, the subcutaneous tissue and skin are closed, and a posterior splint is applied.

Postoperative Management

Crutches are used, and weight-bearing is avoided until 10 to 14 days after surgery when the skin sutures are removed. Therapy and unrestricted weight-bearing are started. If any repairs are performed, running is deferred until 3 months.

Reconstruction of Posterior Tibialis Tendon With FDL Transfer

Technique

1. This procedure proceeds similarly to synovectomy of the tendon sheath. If a tear is identified that leaves less than one-half the diameter of the normal tendon after it has been excised, or if there has been complete rupture of the tendon, reconstruction is performed.
2. The sheath of the flexor digitorum longus (FDL) is entered and opened completely into the midfoot. With tension on the tendon it is cut at the master knot of Henry with scissors. The distal end is let free.
3. The proximal end of the FDL is trimmed and a Bunnell-like stitch placed in it with #1 nonabsorbable suture.
4. A dorsal-to-plantar drill hole is made in the medial pole of the navicular with a ³⁄₆₄ inch drill bit and widened with a small curet, taking care not to fracture the bone.
5. The FDL tendon is then woven through the posterior tibialis tendon three or four times, stoppping at its inferior edge at the level of the navicular.

6. The tendon is passed upward through the drill hole in the navicular and then back onto the woven tendons proximally.

7. The foot is placed in plantarflexion and supination, and the tendon is tied to itself. Multiple stitches of a 0 absorbable suture are placed at each weave of the FDL through the posterior tibialis, at the plantar and dorsal holes in the navicular, and at the site where the tendon is tied back on itself.

8. The tendon sheath is repaired with a running stitch of 2-0 absorbable suture, and the subcutaneous and skin layers are closed separately. A short leg cast is applied with the foot in plantarflexion and supination.

Postoperative Management

The sutures are removed after 10 to 14 days, and another cast is worn until 4 weeks after surgery. A walking cast is then applied with the foot positioned plantigrade and is worn for 4 weeks, after which a walking orthosis is used for an additional 4 weeks. At 12 weeks after surgery protection is removed, and therapy for range of motion, strengthening, and proprioception of the ankle and foot iks started. Return to activity takes 4 to 6 months.

Flexor Hallucis Longus Tendon

Injury to the flexor hallucis longus tendon at the ankle has been recognized primarily in runners and dancers with occurrence reported in a diver and tennis player (Cowell and Elener, 1982; Frey and Shereff, 1988; Hamilton, 1982; McCarroll et al., 1983; Newman and Fowles, 1984; Sammarco and Miller, 1979; Trepman et al., 1995). The flexor hallucis longus tendon (FHL) enters the foot through a fibroosseous tunnel along the posterior ankle. Its superior edge is defined by the posterolateral process of the talus, and it extends inferiorly to the sustentaculum tali on the medial side of the hindfoot. The tendon direction changes from a vertical ori-

entation to horizontal within this tunnel (Mink et al., 1991). As a result, the tendon can become irritated, developing partial intrasubstance tears, that cause it to swell and become tethered (Fig. 5.12).

Clinical Presentation

Pain is present in the posterior ankle between the talus and the Achilles tendon. Deep palpation in this area may reveal tenderness. The pain is typically aggravated by passive motion of the great toe. With significant swelling

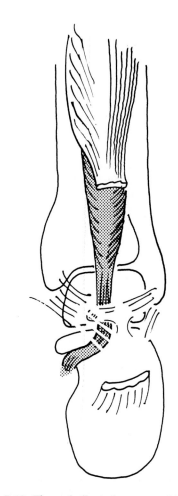

FIGURE 5.12. Flexor hallucis longus and its tendon. The flexor hallucis longus tendon runs in a tunnel along the posterior and medial ankle to the level of the sustentaculum tali. The upper level of the tunnel is defined by the posterior tubercles of the talus.

the tendon may become entrapped and cause triggering, leading to intermittent clawing of the great toe (Cowell and Elener, 1982; Hamilton, 1982, 1993; McCarroll et al., 1983; Newman and Fowles, 1984; Sammarco and Miller, 1979; Trepman et al., 1995). Entrapment can be verified by comparing hallux metatarsophalangeal (MTP) extension with the ankle in the neutral and plantarflexed positions. With entrapment, passive motion of the joint is possible in the plantarflexed position but not when the ankle is held in neutral (Jones, 1993).

Radiography

Routine radiographs are unremarkable, though if they show a coincident os trigonum or large posterior talar process the diagnosis may be misinterpreted. MRI is a useful test for evaluating difficult cases (Mink et al., 1991; Trepman et al., 1995). Fluid can be identified about the tendon in the area of the fibroosseous tunnel from the level of the posterior talus to the sustentaculum tali.

Nonoperative Treatment

The nonoperative treatment is the same as for posterior ankle impingement. Activity limitations and NSAIDs for a short course of 10 to 14 days may provide relief. Immobilization in a short-leg walking cast with an extended toe plate to prevent great toe motion may be helpful as well.

Operative Treatment

For athletes who do not obtain relief with nonoperative methods or those who have persistent triggering of the great toe, release of the fibroosseous tunnel of the flexor hallucis longus tendon is warranted. The medial approach is favored because it allows access to the entire fibroosseous canal. Many case reports suggest that full return of function can be expected after this procedure (Cowell and Elener; 1982; Hamilton, 1982; McCarroll et al., 1983; Newman and Fowles, 1984; Sammarco and Miller,1979; Trepman et al., 1995).

Surgical Release of the FHL Sheath

Technique

1. A general anesthetic is administered and a thigh tourniquet applied. A bump is placed under the opposite hip to facilitate exposure of the medial side of the posterior ankle.
2. A longitudinal curved incision is made in line with the flexor tendons posterior to the medial malleolus. The flexor retinaculum is divided in line with the incision, and the flexor digitorum longus tendon is identified by dorsiflexing the toes. The dissection continues in the interval between the flexor digitorum longus tendon and the posterior tibial artery adjacent to the tendon.
3. With the neurovascular bundle gently retracted posteriorly and the flexor digitorum longus tendon anteriorly, the underlying flexor hallucis longus tendon is seen intimately applied to the posterior ankle. Dorsiflexion of the great toe helps to identify its tendon. The tunnel through which the FHL passes into the foot is defined by the trigonal process.
4. The sheath overlying the tendon is then split in a proximal to distal direction to the level of the sustentaculum tali. The neurovascular bundle should be identified over the course of this dissection to avoid injury to it. The tendon is inspected to identify any longitudinal tear; if present, it is débrided and repaired with a running stitch of 3–0 absorbable suture.
5. The wound is closed in layers, with the flexor retinaculum repaired using 2–0 absorbable sutures. After closing the skin, a well padded posterior splint is applied.

Postoperative Management

No weight-bearing is allowed for 10 to 14 days. The skin sutures are then removed, and weight-bearing is allowed to progress as tolerated. Therapy for local muscle strengthening is started, but training activities should be avoided until 6 weeks after the surgery.

Tibialis Anterior Tendon

The anterior tibialis muscle originates from the proximal tibia and interosseous membrane. It becomes tendinous at the level of the distal tibial metaphysis. The tendon passes in front of the ankle in a straight course underneath the superior extensor retinaculum to attach to the dorsum of the medial cuneiform and base of the first metatarsal. It is the primary dorsiflexor of the ankle and a secondary invertor (Frey and Shereff, 1988). Despite its subcutaneous course, the tendon is rarely injured, probably because it does not change direction against a bony fulcrum and because of its excellent blood supply (Geppert et al., 1993; Trevino and Baumhauer, 1992).

Clinical Presentation

Tendinitis can be due to overuse and has been described due to direct pressure against the subcutaneous tendon by ski boots (Trevino and Baumhauer, 1992). Rupture of the anterior tibialis tendon is an unusual injury that occurs in two distinct populations. The most common presentation is in elderly persons who have an atraumatic rupture. They typically note the insidious onset of a footdrop (Jones, 1993; Ouzounian and Anderson, 1995). The second presentation follows an acute traumatic episode, generally also in older individuals who may be involved in sporting activities, but it can also occur in young athletes (Frey and Shereff, 1988; Ouzounian and Anderson, 1995; Stuart, 1991).

Patients with tendinitis are noted to have tenderness over the course of the tendon and pain with resisted dorsiflexion of the ankle. A rupture can be diagnosed by a visual or palpable defect in the tendon, weakness of ankle dorsiflexion, or footdrop.

Radiography

Routine radiographs are unremarkable. Although the rupture can readily be identified with an MRI scan, the diagnosis should be apparent clinically (Mink et al., 1991; Ouzounian and Anderson, 1995).

Nonoperative Treatment

Tendinitis is treated by activity limitation and NSAIDs. If it is caused by direct pressure against the tendon, the irritant should be relieved.

Operative Treatment

Chronic rupture in the older patient may be satisfactorily treated with a brace, or it may even be left untreated (Bernstein, 1995). In the young patient surgery should be performed. When rupture of the tendon is recognized early, a direct repair is possible (Jones, 1993; Ouzounian and Anderson, 1995; Stuart, 1991; Trevino and Baumhauer, 1992). If the rupture has been unrecognized for several months, reconstruction using extensor hallucis longus tendon transfer or interposition of an extensor digitorum longus tendon graft can be performed, allowing return to recreational activities (Ouzounian and Anderson, 1995).

References

Abraham E, Pankovich AM: Neglected rupture of the achilles tendon. J Bone Joint Surg Am 57:253, 1975

Bernstein RM: Spontaneous rupture of the tibialis anterior tendon. Am J Orthop 24:354–356, 1995

Bosworth DM: Repair of defects in the tendo achilles. J Bone Joint Surg Am 38:111, 1956

Cain MR, Baxter DE: Achilles tendinitis. Foot Ankle 13:482–487, 1992

Carr AJ, Norris SH: The blood supply of the calcaneal tendon. J Bone Joint Surg Br 71: 100–101.

Cetti R, Christensen SE, Ejsted R, et al: Operative versus nonoperative treatment of achilles tendon rupture: a prospective randomized study and review of the literature. Am J Sports Med 21:791–799, 1993

Clancy WG, Neidhart D, Brand RL: Achilles tendonitis in runners: a report of five cases. Am J Sports Med 4:46–56, 1976

Conti SF: Posterior tibial tendon problems in athletes. Orthop Clin North Am 25:109–121, 1994

Copeland SA: Rupture of the achillies tendon: a new clinical test. Ann R Coll Surg Engl 72:270–271, 1990

Cowell HR, Elener V: Bilateral tendonitis of the flexor hallucis longus in a ballet dancer. J Pediatr Orthop 2:582–586, 1982

Frey CC, Shereff MJ: Tendon injuries about the ankle in atheletes. Clin Sports Med 7:103–118, 1988

Frey C, Shereff M, Greenidge N: Vascularity of the posterior tibial tendon. J Bone Joint Surg Am 72:884–888, 1990

Funk DA, Cass JR, Johnson K: Acquired adult flat foot secondary to posterior tibial-tendon pathology. J Bone Joint Surg Am 68:95–102, 1986

Geppert MJ, Sobel M, Hannafin JA: Microvasculature of the tibialis anterior tendon. Foot Ankle 14:261–264, 1993

Hamilton WG: Foot and ankle injuries in dancers. In: Mann RA, Couglin MJ (eds): Surgery of the Foot and Ankle, pp 1241–1277. St. Louis, Mosby, 1993

Hamilton, WG: Stenosing tenosynovitis of the flexor hallucis longus tendon and posterior impingement upon the os trigonum in ballet dancers. Foot Ankle 3:74–80, 1982

Inglis AE, Scott, WN, Sculco TP, et al: Ruptures of the tendo Achilles: an objective assessment of surgical and non-surgical treatment. J Bone Joint Surg Am 58:990–993, 1976

Johnson KA, Strom DE: Tibialis posterior tendon dysfunction. Clin Orthop 239:196–206, 1989

Jones DC: Tendon disorders of the foot and ankle. J Am Acad Orthop Surg 1:87–94, 1993

Kannus P, Jozsa L: Histological changes preceding spontaneous rupture of a tendon: a controlled study of 891 patients. J Bone Joint Surg Am 73:1507–1525, 1991

Kilkelly FX, McHale KA: Acute rupture of the peroneal longus tendon in a runner: a case report and review of the literature. Foot Ankle 15:567–569, 1994

Kleinman M, Gross AE: Achilles tendon rupture following steroid injection. J Bone Joint Surg Am 65:1345–1347, 1983

Krissoff WB, Ferris WD: Runners injuries. Physician Sportsmed 7:55–64, 1979

Kvist M, Jozsa L, Jarvinen MJ, Kvist H: Chronic achilles paratendonitis in athletes: a histological and histochemical study. Pathology 19:1–11, 1987

Lynn TA: Repair of the torn achilles tendon, using the plantaris tendon as a reinforcing membrane. J Bone Joint Surg Am 48:268, 1966

Ma GWC, Griffith TG: Percutaneous repair of acute closed ruptured achilles tendon: a new technique. Clin Orthop 128:247–255, 1977

Maffulli N, Regine R, Angelillo M, et al: Ultra-sound diagnosis of achilles tendon pathology in runners. Br J Sports Med 21, 158–162, 1987

Mahler F, Fritschy D: Partial and complete ruptures of the achilles tendon and local corticosteroid injections. Br J Sports Med 26:7–14, 1992

Mann RA: Biomechanics of the foot and ankle. In: Mann RA, Coughlin MJ (eds): Surgery of the Foot and Ankle, pp 3–43. St. Louis, Mosby, 1993

Mann RA, Holmes GB Jr, Seale KS, et al: Chronic rupture of the achilles tendon: a new technique of repair. J Bone Joint Surg Am 73:214–219, 1991

Mandelbaum BR, Myerson MS, Forster R: Achilles tendon ruptures: a new method of repair, early range of motion, and functional rehabilitation. Am J Sports Med 23:392–395, 1995

Marcus DS, Reicher MA, Kellerhouse LE: Achilles tendon injuries: the role of MR imaging. J Comput Assist Tomogr 13:480–486, 1989

McCarroll JR, Ritter MA, Becker TE: Triggering of the great toe: a case report. Clin Orthop 175:184–185, 1983

Meyer AW: Further evidence of attrition in the human body. Am J Anat 34:241–367, 1924

Mink JH, Deutsch AL, Kerr R: Tendon injuries of the lower extremity: magnetic resonance assessment. Top Magn Reson Imaging 3:23–38, 1991

Monto RR, Moorman CT, Mallon WJ, Nunley JA: Rupture of the posterior tibial tendon associated with closed ankle fracture. Foot Ankle 11:400–403, 1991

Nelen G, Martens M, Burssens A: Surgical treatment of chronic achilles tendinitis. Am J Sports Med 17:754–759, 1989

Newman NM, Fowles JV: A case of "trigger toe." Can J Surg 27:378–379, 1984

Nistor L: Surgical and non-surgical treatment of achilles tendon rupture. J Bone Joint Surg Am 63:394–399, 1981

Ouzounian TJ, Anderson R: Anterior tibial tendon rupture. Foot Ankle 16:406–410, 1995

Peterson DA, Stinson W: Excision of the fractured os peroneum: a report on five patients and review of the literature. Foot Ankle 13:277–281, 1992

Sammarco GJ: Peroneal tendon injuries. Orthop Clin North Am 25:135–145, 1994

Sammarco GJ, DeRaimondo CV: Chronic peroneus brevis tendon lesions. Foot Ankle 9:163–189, 1989

Sammarco GJ, Miller EH: Partial rupture of the

flexor hallucis longus tendon in classical ballet dancers. J Bone Joint Surg Am 61:149–150, 1979

Sarrafian SK: Anatomy of the Foot and Ankle: Descriptive, Topographic, Functional. Philadelphia, Lippincott, 1983

Scheller AD, Kasser JR, Quigley TB: Tendon injuries about the ankle. Orthop Clin North Am 11:801, 1980

Scoli MW: Achilles tendinitis. Orthop Clin North Am 25:177–182, 1994

Skeoch DU: Spontaneous partial subcutaneous ruptures of the tendo achilles: review of the literature and evaluation of 16 involved tendons. Am J Sports Med 9:20–22, 1981

Smart GW, Taunton JE, Clement DB: Achilles tendon disorders in runners—a review. Med Sci Sports Exerc 12:231–243, 1980

Sobel M, Pavlov H, Geppert MJ et al: Painful os peroneum syndrome: a spectrum of conditions responsible for plantar lateral foot pain. Foot Ankle 15:112–124, 1994

Stuart MJ: Traumatic disruption of the anterior tibial tendon while cross-country skiing: a case report. Clin Orthop 281:193–194, 1992

Thompson TC, Doherty JH: Spontaneous rupture of the tendon of the achilles: a new clinical diagnostic test. J Trauma 2:126–129, 1962

Thompson FM, Patterson AH: Rupture of the peroneus longus tendon: report of three cases. J Bone Surg Am 71:293–295, 1989

Trepman E, Mizel MS, Newberg AH: Partial rupture of the flexor hallucis longus tendon in a tennis player: a case report. Foot Ankle 16:227–231, 1995

Trevino S, Baumhauer JF: Tendon injuries of the foot and ankle. Clin Sports Med 11:727–739, 1992

Trevino SG, Gould N, Korson R: Surgical treatment of stenosing tenosynovitis at the ankle. Foot Ankle 2:37–45, 1981

Wapner KL, Pavlok GS, Hecht PJ, et al: Repair of chronic achilles tendon rupture with flexor hallucis longus tendon transfer. Foot Ankle 14:443–449, 1993

White RK, Kraynick BM: Surgical use of the peroneus brevis tendon. Surg Gynecol Obstet 108:117, 1959

Woods L, Leach RE: Posterior tibial tendon rupture in athletic people. Am J Sports Med 19:495–498, 1991

6
Nerve Injuries

Morton's Neuroma

One of the most common causes of forefoot pain is irritation of an interdigital nerve termed Morton's neuroma. The typical symptoms were first described in 1876 by Thomas Morton, and in 1940 Betts identified a neuroma as the cause of this pain. The syndrome has classically referred to neurogenic pain in the ball of the foot centered between the third and fourth toes.

Morton's neuroma is caused by irritation of the interdigital nerve as it passes under the transverse metatarsal ligament (Fig. 6.1) (Graham and Graham, 1984; Graham et al., 1981; Mann and Reynolds, 1983). During the last stage of stance in the gait cycle, weight is transferred onto the ball of the foot and the toes dorsiflex. The interdigital nerve is squeezed between the plantar aspect of the foot below and the edge of the intermetatarsal ligament above, leading to the development of swelling and fibrosis in the area within and about the nerve at the level of the ligament.

The common digital nerve to the third interspace receives contributions from the medial and lateral plantar nerves, which may produce a tethering effect in this interspace (Jones and Klenerman, 1984). It is also the border of the relatively rigid medial three rays and the relatively mobile lateral two rays, and the digital nerve within this space may be subject to a shearing stress.

Morton's neuroma is a common cause of forefoot pain in the general population. It probably occurs in all sporting populations but has been reported primarily in runners and dancers.

Clinical Presentation

Patients complain of pain in the ball of the foot that is worse with tight shoes and weight-bearing and is relieved by rest. The pain is variably described as burning, stabbing, or a sensation of "standing on a pebble" under the ball of the foot. Symptoms usually develop insidiously, and it is rare that an acute episode is described.

The third interspace is the usual site of Morton's neuroma, but the second interspace is also involved in a significant number of cases (Mann and Reynolds, 1983). The first and fourth are only rarely involved. The occurrence of simultaneous neuromas in multiple interspaces is rare (Thompson and Deland, 1993). If pain occurs across multiple areas, other etiologies must be considered.

A careful examination differentiates tenderness in the interspace from metatarsophalangeal (MTP) joint tenderness. A fullness may be appreciated on palpating the interspace. The pain of a Morton's neuroma can be amplified by palpating the interspace between the thumb and index finger with one hand while simultaneously compressing the forefoot with pressure on the first and fifth metatarsal heads with the other hand. This maneuver may also elicit a palpable or even

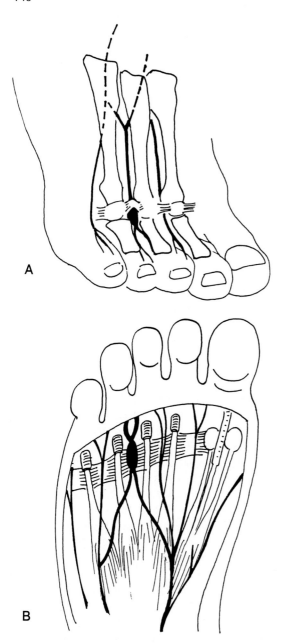

FIGURE 6.1. Morton's neuroma. (A) Anterior view of the foot showing a neuroma in the nerve to the third web space. The neuroma lies underneath the transverse metatarsal ligament. (B) Plantar view of the foot showing the same neuroma. Note the contributions to this nerve from both the medial and lateral plantar nerves.

audible click, termed Mulder's click. In cases where the diagnosis is unclear, selective injections of local anesthetic into the interspace

or the adjacent MTP can be used to identify the origin of the pain.

Radiography

Radiographs are obtained to exclude other pathology, such as a metatarsal stress fracture or abnormality of the MTP joint. The diagnosis is determined from the history and physical examination.

Nonoperative Treatment

A shoe with a narrow toebox "squeezes" the metatarsal heads together, irritating the digital nerve; and elevated heels increase dorsiflexion at the MTP joints. Therefore the first step of treatment is to wear shoes that are flat and have a wide toebox. A HAPAD placed proximal to the MTP joints of the involved interspace transfers plantar pressure proximally and limit pressure in the area of the neuroma. It may also limit dorsiflexion of the involved MTP joints. Stiffening of the sole in the forefoot can also decrease MTP joint motion. Conversely, orthotic devices that extend from the heel only up to the ball of the foot may increase dorsiflexion at the MTP joints and lead to increased nerve irritation.

Corticosteroid injection into the interspace may give long-standing or even permanent relief (Greenfield et al., 1984).

1. A 25 gauge 1.5 inch needle is attached to a 3 ml syringe filled with 1% lidocaine without epinephrine and inserted into the dorsum of the foot between the metatarsal heads of the involved interspace. The needle is slowly advanced while injecting the local anesthetic until is contacts the plantar aspect of the foot. It is then withdrawn a distance of approximately 1 cm and the syringe removed from the needle.
2. A 1.0 ml syringe filled with a corticosteroid solution is attached to the needle and the steroid injected into the interspace. Maintaining the position of the needle, the lidocaine only syringe is reattached. As the needle is withdrawn, local anesthetic is continuously injected, a maneuver that

prevents introduction of steroid into the skin or subcutaneous tissue.

Operative Treatment

When conservative treatment is not successful, surgery should be considered. It is an outpatient operation that yields good pain relief in approximately 80% of patients (Johnson et al., 1988; Mann and Reynaolds, 1983), although a significant number of patients continue to be symptomatic after surgery.

Improper web space selection or misdiagnosis of an MTP joint problem as a Morton's neuroma are causes of surgical failure. The formation of a painful stump neuroma is another (Johnson et al., 1988). If the cut end of the nerve does not retract proximally into soft tissue, the resulting stump neuroma may continue to be irritated and cause persistent pain that the athlete perceives as similar to the preoperative pain. There are multiple fine plantar-directed branches of the interdigital nerve that can act to tether the nerve and prevent retraction after neuroma resection (Amis et al., 1992).

When pain persists after excision of the neuroma, the nonoperative treatments should be retried. Additionally, formal physical therapy can provide desensitization by massage of the scar and interspace. Contrast baths and the use of transcutaneous electrical nerve stimulation (TENS) units are often helpful for treating postoperative pain.

The nonoperative treatment should be used for an adequate time before considering a second operation. Repeat excision is done through a plantar approach, as this approach allows better access to the more proximal nerve (Beskin and Baxter, 1988).

Excision of Primary Morton's Neuroma

A primary Morton's neuroma is excised through a dorsal incision at the base of the appropriate web space.

Technique

1. Under tourniquet control, a 3 cm longitudinal incision is made beginning at the base of the identified web space. Hemostasis by electrocautery is important to allow visualization of the nerve. After dissecting through the subcutaneous tissue, the interspace is entered.
2. Upward pressure is manually applied to the ball of the foot, which brings the neuroma into view in the interspace. It is grasped with a small clamp, and the overlying intermetatarsal ligament just proximal to it is cut with tenotomy scissors.
3. The scissors are then used to separate the proximal nerve from its accompanying artery. With distal traction through the clamp the nerve is resected at the highest level. The distal limbs of the nerve are then resected and the specimen sent for histologic confirmation.
4. Hemostasis is meticulously obtained after tourniquet deflation, and the wound is closed in layers. A soft dressing is applied.

Postoperative Management

Immediate weight-bearing is allowed with a postoperative shoe. The sutures are removed at 10 to 14 days, and shoewear is advanced. Athletic activities are avoided for 4 weeks after surgery.

Excision of Recurrent Morton's Neuroma

Reoperation for failed Morton's neuroma surgery is done through a plantar approach (Fig. 6.2). It is technically easier if the patient is in the prone position.

Technique

1. After tourniquet inflation, the heads of the metatarsals bordering the involved interdigital nerve are palpated and marked. A 3 to 4 cm longitudinal incision is made starting between the metatarsal heads and extending proximally. It continues through the subcutaneous tissue and the distal extent of the plantar fascia, which has multiple nonuniform tracts at this level.
2. The nerve is identified proximally, as it lies superficial to the tendons of the flexor

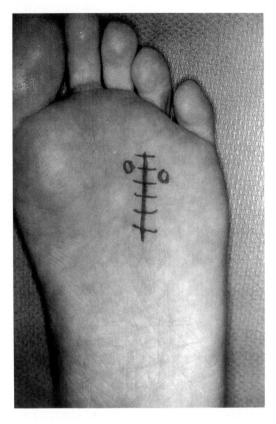

FIGURE 6.2. Plantar incision to remove a recurrent Morton's neuroma.

digitorum longus. It is traced distally to verify that it is directed to the proper interspace. It may be dissected distally with tenotomy scissors to identify the site of previous excision where the stump neuroma has formed.

3. The nerve should be resected as far proximally as possible to ensure that the next stump neuroma that forms is in a well padded area of the midfoot.

4. The wound is closed in layers and a soft dressing applied.

Postoperative Management

The patient is kept non-weight-bearing for 2 weeks, at which point the skin sutures are removed and weight-bearing is advanced as tolerated. Athletic activities should be avoided until 6 weeks after surgery.

Tarsal Tunnel Syndrome

Tarsal tunnel syndrome is defined as entrapment of the posterior tibial nerve in its tunnel as it passes posterior to the medial malleolus to enter the foot (Cimino, 1990). It is analogous to carpal tunnel syndrome, although it occurs much less commonly. The syndrome was first described in 1960 with the terminology coined by Keck in 1962.

Anatomy

The posterior tibial nerve originates from the sciatic nerve and enters the deep posterior compartment of the leg between the two heads of the gastrocnemius. Coursing between the soleus and posterior tibialis muscle, it descends the leg to the ankle. It terminates in three branches in the tarsal tunnel, the medial and lateral plantar nerves and the calcaneal branch.

The medial plantar nerve provides sensation to the plantar medial aspect of the foot, extending from the great toe to the medial half of the fourth toe. The lateral plantar nerve provides sensation from the fourth toe laterally. The medial plantar nerve innervates the abductor hallucis, flexor brevi, and first lumbrical. The lateral nerve's motor innervation includes the abductor digiti quinti, interossei, adductor hallucis, and second to fifth lumbricals. The calcaneal branch provides sensation to the heel pad.

The roof of the tarsal tunnel is formed by the flexor retinaculum, also called the laciniate ligament, which is a fan-shaped structure that attaches anteriorly to the medial malleolus. The retinaculum spreads posteroinferiorly, attaching to the lateral wall of the calcaneus and the superior border of the abductor hallucis fascia. Superiorly, it extends 10 cm proximal to the tip of the malleolus. It has septated attachments to the sheaths of the posterior tibialis, flexor digitorum, and flexor hallucis longus tendons.

Etiology

Tarsal tunnel syndrome occurs when the contents of the tunnel are compressed intrinsically or extrinsically (Cimino, 1990). Space-occupying lesions account for approximately one-half of the cases of tarsal tunnel syndrome. Ganglions, varicosities, lipomas, and neurilemomas have been associated with tarsal tunnel syndrome. Direct trauma to the posterior tibial nerve in the tarsal tunnel can be caused by ill-fitting ski boots. The syndrome has been reported in runners, dancers, and mountain climbers. Repetitive dorsiflexion has been proposed as the cause in this latter group of athletes. In the remaining patients no precise etiology has been identified. The symptoms may be caused by a hypertrophic abductor hallucis muscle or thickened fascia that compresses the plantar nerves.

Clinical Findings

The patient typically describes an insidious onset of symptoms in the sensory distribution of the involved nerves. It may involve one, two, or all three branches of the posterior tibial nerve but usually not the calcaneal branch alone. Intermittent paresthesias, dysesthesias, or anesthesia in the plantar aspect of the foot are described, and there may be proximal radiation of pain. Rest pain is uncommon; and because sensory nerves are smaller and more sensitive to ischemia, motor findings are also uncommon. With long-standing entrapment, intrinsic weakness demonstrated by clawing of the toes or abductor hallucis atrophy may be seen, but it is unusual.

In affected patients, percussion along the course of the posterior tibial nerve in the tarsal tunnel can reproduce symptoms (percussion sign). Manual compression of the tarsal tunnel for 60 seconds may also reproduce symptoms. Finally, heel eversion or inversion can alter the shape of the tarsal tunnel enough to produce symptoms in some patients (Cimino, 1990).

Electrodiagnostic Tests

Electromyography and measurements of nerve conduction velocity are useful for diagnosing tarsal tunnel syndrome. These tests are routinely performed for any patient suspected of having tarsal tunnel syndrome. Electrodiagnostic tests are reliable for the tibial nerve and the plantar nerves but are not useful for evaluating the calcaneal branch.

Posterior tibial nerve conduction velocity is measured to exclude the possibility of peripheral neuropathy. The distal motor latencies of the medial and lateral plantar nerves have been the standard tests for diagnosing tarsal tunnel syndrome. Increases in the terminal latency of the medial plantar nerve above 6.2 ms and the lateral plantar nerve above 7.0 ms have been considered abnormal, although variability occurs (Cimino, 1990). The distal motor latencies give a false negative result in 45% of cases, and a better test is the sensory distal latency, which is positive in 90% of patients with tarsal tunnel syndrome. This test battery is similar to the evaluation for carpal tunnel syndrome, where sensory conduction studies are more sensitive than motor studies.

Electromyography and nerve conduction tests are performed bilaterally in the patient with suspected tarsal tunnel syndrome. None of these tests, however, is definitive. It must be emphasized that these studies are done in the static situation and so often do not identify a nerve entrapment that occurs transiently during activity. Although sensory latency appears to be the most sensitive test, it nonetheless yields a significant number of false negative results. Therefore whereas a positive result may be confirmatory, a negative result does not preclude the diagnosis.

Nonoperative Treatment

The treatment of tarsal tunnel syndrome depends on the etiology. Athletes may do well with a short course of activity restriction or immobilization, a nonsteroidal antiinflammatory medication (NSAID), or steroid injection. Mixed results have been obtained with orthotic prescription. One report found orthotic devices to be helpful in patients in whom hypermobile valgus hindfeet is the cause of tarsal tunnel syndrome. In the athlete with normal foot structure, a soft orthotic insert may alter the geometry of the tarsal tunnel during activity. Oral NSAIDs and steroid injection may reduce inflammation about the nerve and decrease swelling.

Operative Treatment

Surgical decompression is the treatment of choice for space-occupying lesions. A review of 24 reports totaling 122 patients treated surgically found that 91% had complete resolution or only mild residual symptoms (Cimino, 1990).

Tarsal Tunnel Release

Technique

The technique is shown in Figures 6.3 and 6.4.

1. A general anesthetic is preferred, and a thigh tourniquet is used. The patient is positioned supine with a bump placed underneath the contralateral hip to facilitate visualization of the medial hindfoot.
2. An 8 to 10 cm gently curving longitudinal incision is made following the course of the posterior tibial nerve posterior to the medial malleolus to a point 1 cm inferior to the medial pole of the navicular.
3. The flexor retinaculum is divided, beginning proximally and extending to the abductor hallucis muscle fascia. The calcaneal branch or branches extend posteriorly

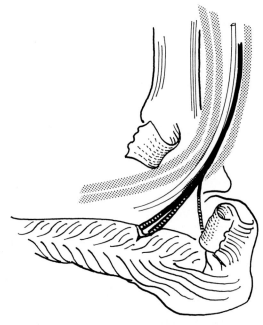

FIGURE 6.3. Tarsal tunnel release. The laciniate ligament (medial retinaculum) has been divided to show the relation between the neurovascular and tendinous structures in the tarsal canal.

and can be protected by keeping the dissection anterior to the medial and lateral branches. The posterior tibial artery must be carefully dissected free from the nerve, which lies posteriorly.

4. The medial and lateral plantar nerves are followed as they travel deep to the abductor hallucis muscle. The dorsal fascia of

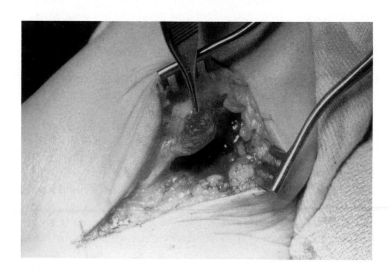

FIGURE 6.4. Tarsal tunnel syndrome caused by a schwannoma of the posterior tibial nerve.

this muscle is divided, as it can compress the underlying nerves.

5. After completely releasing the nerve and removing any identifiable space occupying lesion, the wound is irrigated and closed. The muscle fascia is left unrepaired, as is the flexor retinaculum. The subcutaneous layer is closed with interrupted stitches of 2–0 absorbable suture and the skin is closed with interrupted stitches of 3–0 non-absorbable suture. Steroids should not be injected into the wound, as wound healing can be impaired.

Postoperative Management

The patient is kept non-weight-bearing for 3 to 4 weeks. The skin sutures are removed at 10 to 14 days and range of motion and strengthening exercises are started. Shoewear is advanced and athletic activities can be resumed as tolerated.

Peroneal Nerve Compression

Deep Peroneal Nerve Entrapment

Entrapment of the deep peroneal nerve is also called anterior tarsal tunnel syndrome (Borges et al., 1981; Dellon, 1990). It is much less common than tarsal tunnel syndrome. Pain is located over the dorsum of the foot and in the first web space.

Anatomy

The deep peroneal nerve passes through the anterior compartment of the leg, innervating these muscles and traveling with the anterior tibial artery. It enters the ankle underneath the extensor retinaculum. It then divides into a medial branch, which continues distally with the dorsalis pedis artery and provides sensation to the first web space, and a lateral branch, which innervates the extensor digitorum brevis muscle.

Clinical Presentation

Entrapment of the deep peroneal nerve can occur as the nerve passes under the inferior extensor retinaculum at the ankle. Other causes include compression against dorsal osteophytes of the tarsal bones and shoewear that is tight over the dorsum of the foot (Fig. 6.5). The athlete complains of aching over the dorsum of the foot with numbness or pain in the first web space (Dellon, 1990).

If the lateral branch of the nerve is involved, there is discernible extensor brevis atrophy. Medial branch entrapment causes a sensory deficit in the first web space. Percussion along the nerve can identify the site of entrapment, as noted by increased sensitivity.

Electrodiagnostic Tests

Electrodiagnostic studies of the branch to the extensor digitorum brevis may show an increased distal motor latency, although the proximal nerve conduction velocity is normal. EMG findings of chronic denervation in the extensor brevis is a diagnostic finding. However, a normal EMG does not preclude the diagnosis of nerve entrapment, particularly if the symptoms appear only with activity.

Nonoperative Treatment

Nonoperative treatment involves shoe modification to prevent compression over the dorsum of the foot and oral antiinflammatory

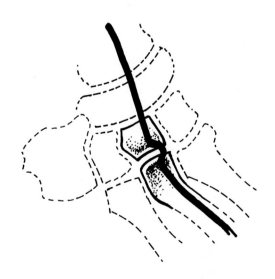

FIGURE 6.5. Compression of the peroneal nerve. The deep peroneal nerve can be compressed between the shoe and an osteophyte at the metatarsal cuneiform joint.

medication. Additionally, local injection of steroid into an identified area of tenderness along the nerve can be useful.

Operative Treatment

Surgery is indicated for persistent symptoms and is directed at decompressing the nerve by releasing the tight extensor retinaculum or removing dorsal osteophytes (or both).

Technique

1. Appropriate anesthesia and a thigh tourniquet are used. A 5 cm longitudinal incision is made over the dorsum of the hindfoot, extending distally from the ankle joint.
2. The inferior extensor retinaculum is identified and sharply divided. The deep peroneal nerve is then identified in the interval between the extensor hallucis longus and the extensor digitorum longus tendons.
3. The nerve is followed distally, being careful not to damage the lateral branch to the extensor digitorum brevis at the proximal extent of the wound.
4. If there are any osteophytes contributing to the nerve entrapment, they are identified, the nerve gently retracted, the periosteum over the prominence split, and the bone removed with a rongeur or osteotome. The base of the bone is smoothed and the periosteum closed over it.
5. The subcutaneous layer is closed with interrupted 2-0 absorbable suture and the skin closed with interrupted 3-0 nonabsorbable suture. A soft dressing is applied.

Postoperative Management

The patient is kept non-weight-bearing for 10 to 14 days. The skin sutures are then removed, and weight-bearing in a shoe is started. Activities may be resumed 3 to 4 weeks after surgery.

Superficial Peroneal Nerve Entrapment

Entrapment of the superficial peroneal nerve is uncommon but may occur where the nerve passes through the fascia as it exits the lateral

compartment of the leg. Exertional anterolateral compartment syndrome and muscle herniation through a fascial defect have been associated with this entrapment. The athlete complains of pain at the site of the fascial defect, where there is often a noticeable bulge. There may also be pain or numbness appreciated on the dorsum of the foot. The symptoms usually resolve soon after activity is halted.

The superficial peroneal nerve is also at risk of injury during ankle arthroscopy. Placement of the anterolateral portal lies over the course of the nerve at the level of the ankle joint. Unless care is taken to identify and protect the nerve it may be partially or completely transected, leading to a painful neuroma or dysesthesia (Fig. 6.6).

Anatomy

The superficial peroneal nerve is a branch of the common peroneal nerve, which innervates the peroneus longus and brevis muscles in the lateral compartment. It then exits the fascia about 10 cm proximal to the ankle, becoming subcutaneous. It branches into the medial and intermediate dorsal cutaneous nerves proximal to the ankle, which supply sensation over the dorsum of the foot with the exception of the first web space.

Physical Examination

Physical examination may reveal a bulge at the site of a fascial defect that can be demon

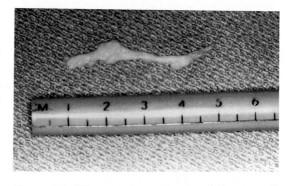

FIGURE 6.6. Neuroma in continuity of the superficial peroneal nerve that resulted from placing an anterolateral portal for ankle arthroscopy. Neurectomy was performed.

strated better by resisted ankle dorsiflexion. The athlete, after running a short distance to produce symptoms, is reexamined to see if the muscle herniates through the fascial defect. The mass may be tender with a positive percussion sign causing radiation over the dorsum of the foot. Electrodiagnostic studies are not useful for evaluating of this entrapment.

Nonoperative Treatment

Oral NSAIDs can be used for a short course. A steroid injection into the area of muscle herniation may relieve swelling about the nerve and provide symptomatic improvement. If these measures are not successful, surgical decompression by partial fasciotomy of the lateral compartment is performed.

Operative Treatment

Partial fasciotomy of the anterior compartment of the leg is performed.

Technique

1. Under tourniquet control, the fascial defect is identified by palpation, and a longitudinal incision is made extending from 1 cm proximal to 5 cm distal.
2. With careful dissection the nerve is identified as it exits the defect. The nerve is protected, and the fascia of the compartment is split proximally and distally to release it.
3. The subcutaneous layer is closed with interrupted 2-0 absorbable suture and the skin closed with interrupted 3-0 nonabsorbable suture. A soft dressing is applied.

Postoperative Management

The patient is kept non-weight-bearing for 10 to 14 days. The skin sutures are then removed, and weight-bearing in a shoe is started. Activities may be resumed 3 to 4 weeks after surgery.

Sural Nerve Entrapment

The sural nerve is a branch of the tibial nerve that accompanies the small saphenous vein.

It provides sensation to the calf, lateral heel, and lateral border of the foot. Entrapment of the sural nerve is rare, probably because it is protected over its course by subcutaneous tissue and does not pass under restraining fascial edges or against bones. Cases of entrapment can occur against a fracture of the lateral malleolus, tarsal bone, or fifth metatarsal that healed with a bony prominence or against an adjacent ganglion. A tight shoe with a firm lateral counter occasionally causes irritation of the nerve, simulating entrapment.

Clinical Presentation

The athlete has pain or paresthesias (or both) in the distribution of the sural nerve and may have a percussion sign over the site of entrapment. There may be a history of prior ankle or lateral foot fracture. Ankle flexion and supination of the foot may reproduce the symptoms by placing the nerve on stretch.

Nonoperative Treatment

Nonoperative treatment includes shoe modification to avoid pressure over the area of entrapment and posting of the lateral heel to maintain a valgus hindfoot position. Rest and oral antiinflammatory medication can be used with limited efficacy. A steroid injection may be helpful if a specific site of nerve irritation can be identified.

Operative Treatment

Surgery is performed to remove the object that is causing compression of the nerve in recalcitrant cases.

References

Amis JA, Siverhus SW, Liwnicz BH: An anatomic basis for recurrence after Morton's neuroma excision. Foot Ankle 13:153–156, 1992

Beskin JL, Baxter DE: Recurrent pain following interdigital neurectomy—a plantar approach. Foot Ankle 9:34–39, 1988

Borges LF, Halle HM, Selkie DJ: The anterior tarsal tunnel syndrome: report of two cases. J Neurosurg 54:89, 1981

Cimino WR: Tarsal tunnel syndrome: review of the literature. Foot Ankle 11:47–52,1990

Dellon AL: Deep peroneal nerve entrapment on the dorsum of the foot. Foot Ankle 11:73–80, 1990

Garfin S, Mubarak SJ, Owen CA: Exertional anterolateral compartment syndrome. J Bone Joint Surg 59A:404–405, 1977

Gessini L, Jandols B, Pietrangel A: The anterior tarsal tunnel syndrome. J Bone Joint Surg. 66A:786–787, 1984

Gould N, Trevino S: Sural nerve entrapment by avulsion fracture at the base of the fifth metatarsal bone. Foot Ankle 2:153–155, 1981

Graham CE, Graham DM: Morton's Neuroma: a microscopic evaluation. Foot Ankle 5:150–153, 1984

Graham CE, Johnson KA, Ilstrup DM: The intermetatarsal nerve: a microscopic evaluation. Foot Ankle 2:150–152, 1981

Greenfield J, Rea J, Ilfeld FW: Morton's interdigital neuroma: indications for treatment by local injections versus surgery. Clin Orthop 185:142–144, 1984

Johnson JE, Johnson KA, Unni KK: Persistent pain after excision of an interdigital neuroma. J Bone Joint Surg Am 70:651–657, 1988

Jones JR, Klenerman L: A study of the communicating branch between the medial and lateral plantar nerves. Foot Ankle 4:313–315, 1984

Mann RA, Reynolds JC: Interdigital neuroma—a critical clinical analysis. Foot Ankle 3:238–243, 1983

Pringle RM, Protheroe K, Mukherjee SK: Entrapment neuropathy of the sural nerve: J Bone Joint Surg 56B:465–000, 1974

Sarrafian S: Anatomy of the Foot and Ankle. Philadelphia, Lippincott, 1993

Schon LC: Tarsal tunnel release. In Myerson M (ed). Current Therapy Foot and Ankle Surgery. St. Louis, Mosby (Year-book), pp 173–176, 1993

Styf J: Diagnosis of exercise induced pain in the anterior aspect of the lower leg. Am J Sports Med 16:165–169, 1988

Thompson FM, Deland JT: Occurrence of two interdigital neuromas in one foot. Foot Ankle 14:15–17, 1993

7
Skin and Nails

The skin is the largest organ of the body. Enclosing the other tissues it acts as a protective barrier that maintains a stable internal chemical environment. The plantar skin of the foot, as well, provides protection from the high pressures of weight-bearing. Skin blocks the invasion of infectious organisms. Constriction and dilation of blood vessels in the skin and the sweat mechanism are important factors in the regulation of body temperature. The skin provides a large sensory interface with the external world through which varied information is input to the brain, including temperature, pressure, pain, pleasure, and position.

The skin is comprised of two layers, the dermis and epidermis (AAOS, 1991) (Fig. 7.1). The dermis rests on the subcutaneous fat and contains various specialized structures. Sweat glands in the dermis produce sweat that exits through pores in the epidermis, cooling the body as it evaporates. Sebaceous glands produce oily sebum that acts as waterproofing for the epidermis and keeps it supple. Hair follicles produce hair, one hair per follicle. Piloerection causes the hair to stand up from the skin in response to cold temperature or fright. Blood vessels in the dermis are under neuroregulatory control and participate in temperature regulation. When the core body temperature rises, the blood vessels dilate, allowing more heat to be carried to the large surface area and dissipated. Conversely, a drop in the core temperature causes constriction of the dermal ves-

sels. Finally, there are specialized nerve endings such as pacinian corpuscles, which sense pressure, and glomus bodies, which sense temperature in the dermis.

The epidermis is composed of several layers. The deepest is the germinal layer, which contains the skin pigment and is constantly producing new cells. These cells gradually rise to the surface, dying along the way. The sebum produced in the dermis helps hold these cells together, providing a watertight barrier. The outermost layer of dead cells is constantly being sloughed and replaced from underneath.

The plantar skin is different from the hairy skin found on the rest of the body because it must absorb the shock of weight-bearing (Sammarco, 1982). The underlying heel pad has a unique structure, composed of a meshwork of fibrous septae that enclose pockets of fat in a closed-cell configuration that provides cushioning (Jahss et al., 1992). Sensory feedback protects the skin from abrasion injuries, allowing barefoot activities (Robbins et al., 1993).

Specific Skin Disorders

Corns and Plantar Callus

Corns and calluses are hyperkeratotic areas that develop in response to increased pressure in the skin (McNerney, 1990). They are an attempt by the skin to form a better

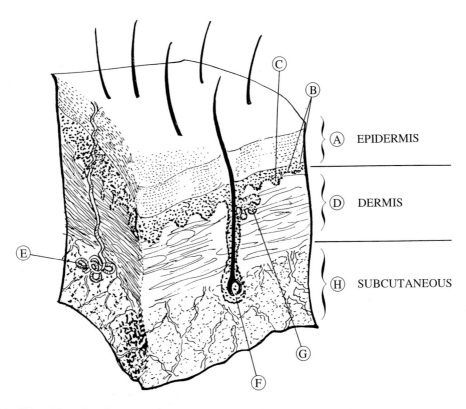

FIGURE 7.1. Skin. The skin has two layers, epidermis and dermis, that lie above the subcutaneous fat. The major structures lie in the dermis.

A, epidermis; B, germinal layer; C, pigment granules; D, dermis; E, sweat gland; F, hair follicle; G, sebaceous gland; H, subcutaneous fat.

protective layer (Sammarco, 1982). Typically, the term "corn" describes a lesion on the toe, whereas "callus" is used for the bottom or sides of the foot. An "end corn" is found on the tip of a toe and a "hard corn" over the dorsum of the proximal (PIP) or distal (DIP) interphalangeal joint. The fourth and fifth toes may have a hard corn on the lateral side of an interphalangeal joint (Fig. 7.2). These spots are the usual areas where bony prominences rub against the shoes. They are common with hammertoe and clawtoe deformities but can occur in feet with normal architecture if ill-fitting shoes are worn.

"Soft corns" develop at the base of the web space between the lesser toes, usually the fourth and fifth, where prominent phalangeal condyles rub against each other and catch the overlying skin between them (Fig. 7.3). The base of the web space is an intertriginous area that is easily macerated. Soft corns may lead to ulceration and abscess formation in the web space.

A plantar callus may be diffuse or well localized, and if painful it is called an intractable plantar keratosis (IPK) (Fig. 7.4). These lesions develop when there is pressure concentration under the metatarsal heads or sesamoids (Fig. 7.5). Clawtoes and a cavus foot tend to have increased pressure over a wide area and lead to diffuse callus formation. A dislocated metatarsophalangeal (MTP), single hammertoe, metatarsal fracture, or sesamoid fracture is more likely to be

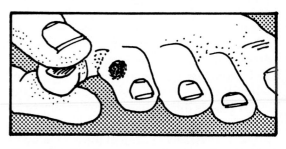

FIGURE 7.2. Hard corn over the lateral condyle of the fourth toe PIP joint.

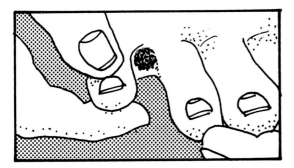

FIGURE 7.3. Soft corn at the base of the fourth web space.

associated with an IPK. In some instances an abnormal plantar condyle under a metatarsal head can cause an IPK to form.

A single hyperkeratotic lesion under the ball of the foot may be a plantar wart, and it is important to differentiate between this lesion and an IPK. An IPK should be directly under a bone prominence. Examination of the papillary lines in the skin (the lines that make the fingerprint) shows that they pass through a corn undisturbed but pass around a plantar wart. If a scalpel is used to carefully pare the layers of the lesion, a corn shows a hard, translucent center called the core. When trimming a wart, multiple small blood vessels are seen end-on and appear as dark dots. Further paring causes these vessels to bleed, and the bleeding may be profuse.

When evaluating corns and calluses, the underlying cause should be determined and treated with the methods described elsewhere. Nonoperative measures are aimed at relieving the external pressure against the foot, and surgical treatment involves removing the prominence in the foot.

Nonoperative Management

An adequate toebox that does not rub against the toes is the first thing to consider. HAPADs decrease the pressure under the metatarsal heads and provide a simple, inexpensive way to relieve plantar calluses (Fig. 7.6). (Hayda et al., 1994; Holmes and Timmerman, 1990).

The pressure on an end corn can be relieved by use of a toe crest to elevate the end of the toe from the insole. A sponge cap that fits over the end of the toe may provide

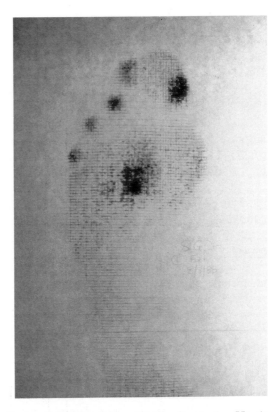

FIGURE 7.5. Intractable plantar keratosis. Harris mat ink impression of the IPK, which is under the second metatarsal head. There is also increased pressure demonstrated under the medial side of the great toe.

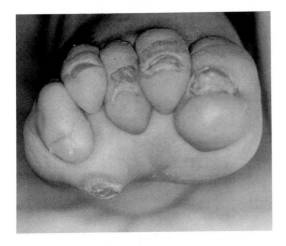

FIGURE 7.4. Intractable plantar keratosis under the fourth metatarsal head.

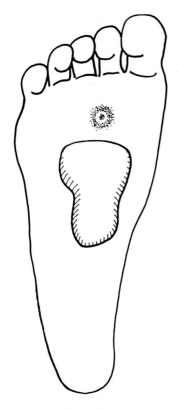

FIGURE 7.6. HAPAD treatment for plantar callus. The HAPAD is placed on the insole just proximal to the callus in order to alleviate pressure on the lesion.

additional cushioning. A corn over an interphalangeal joint may also be treated with a toe crest or sponge pad. Pads or lambs wool placed between the toes can separate them enough to eliminate a hard corn caused by condyles of adjacent toes rubbing together and can treat a soft corn at the base of a web space.

A corn that erodes through the skin to form an ulcer requires wound care in addition to relief of the pressure that caused the corn to form. Soaking the foot in warm, soapy water for 5 to 10 minutes at least twice a day can keep the ulcer clean. A topical antibiotic salve should be applied to the ulcer after soaking.

Diffuse calluses on the bottom of the foot can be kept in check by use of a pumice stone or other mildly abrasive tool. The pumice is used after a shower or bath has softened the skin. Daily use prevents buildup of significant callus that may become tender.

The pumice stone can also be used on

IPKs, but these discrete lesions may continue to be painful even with daily débridement. A scalpel can be used to intermittently pare the IPK and remove the hard central core (Cracchiolo, 1982). This treatment is then followed by daily use of the pumice stone. Diffuse calluses and corns on the toes are usually not amenable to significant débridement with a scalpel.

Technique

1. A #10 scalpel is first used to pare the outer layers of hyperkeratotic skin from an IPK (Fig. 7.7A). Local anesthesia is not necessary, as the lesion is insensate. It is important to work carefully and gradually with tangential cuts, not being overly aggres-

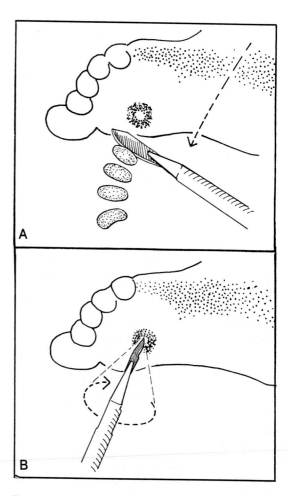

FIGURE 7.7. Trimming a plantar callus. (A) Callus is first pared with a no. 10 scalpel. (B) Central core is then excised with a no. 15 scalpel.

sive with each stroke, thereby decreasing the chance that normal skin is cut, which can cause bleeding and discomfort.

2. After trimming the lesion back to a shallow crater the tip of a #15 scalpel is used to carve out the central core of the callus (Fig. 7.7B). The scalpel tip cuts a cone-shaped segment from the remaining lesion, again being careful not to cut deep into the bleeding dermis.

3. Daily use of a pumice stone after bathing or showering delays the return of the corn. There should be immediate relief from the trimming and no time lost from athletic activities.

Operative Treatment

As with other lesions in the forefoot, surgery is indicated for corns and calluses when the nonoperative treatment has been unsuccessful. Corns over the dorsum of the interphalangeal joints are treated with the methods described for hammertoes. Hard corns between toes are due to pressure from phalangeal condyles of adjacent toes and can usually be relieved by phalangeal condylectomy on one of the toes. Soft corns at the base of a web space are treated with syndactylization of the toes to the level of the PIP without the need for bone excision.

Intractable plantar keratoses should also be treated by first addressing the underlying pathology. Plantar condylectomy of the metatarsal head removes the prominence causing the pressure lesion. However, it involves entering the MTP joint and can lead to stiffness. Proximal and midshaft osteotomies have been advocated, usually with internal fixation; the amount of elevation of the metatarsal head may be difficult to judge (Sclamberg and Lorenz, 1983). The Wolf distal metatarsal osteotomy avoids entering the joint, achieves controlled elevation of the metatarsal head, and effectively relieves IPKs (Leventen and Pearson, 1990; Wolf, 1973).

Condylectomy for Hard Corn

Technique

1. Appropriate anesthesia and a tourniquet are used. An elliptical incision is made along the side of the toe centered on the corn to be is removed. The periosteum is then incised in line with the skin incision and elevated dorsal and plantar.

2. The condyle is exposed and removed with a small rongeur. The sides of the rongeur are used rather than the tip to ensure that bone resection is smooth rather than jagged.

3. The periosteum is closed over the bone with 3–0 absorbable suture and the skin closed with simple nonabsorbable suture.

Postoperative Management. After application of dressings, weight-bearing is allowed with a postoperative shoe. The sutures are removed after 10 to 14 days, and return to full activities is allowed immediately.

Syndactylization for Soft Corn

Surgical Technique

1. Under tourniquet control, use a marking pen to make a longitudinal scribe along one side of the web space, beginning at the base and extending to just proximal to the PIP (Fig. 7.8A). The two toes are then aligned and pressed together, causing the mark to be partially transferred to the adjacent toe. This method marks the incision on both toes and ensures that the toes will be normally aligned after closure.

2. The two marked incisions are opened, and a third limb of the incision is opened by extending the wound longitudinally from the base of the web space between the metatarsals dorsally for 1 cm. The corn is then excised and small flaps developed (Fig. 7.8B).

3. The plantar halves of the wound on each toe are then closed together with a 3–0 absorbable suture using simple stitches so the knots are superior, which has the effect of burying them (FIg. 7.8C).

4. The dorsal wound is closed with 4–0 nonabsorbable suture using simple stitiches (Fig. 7.8D). It is easiest to begin distally and extend proximally until the entire wound is closed. For additional stability a single, simple nonabsorbable stitch can be placed by the ends of the toes, holding them together.

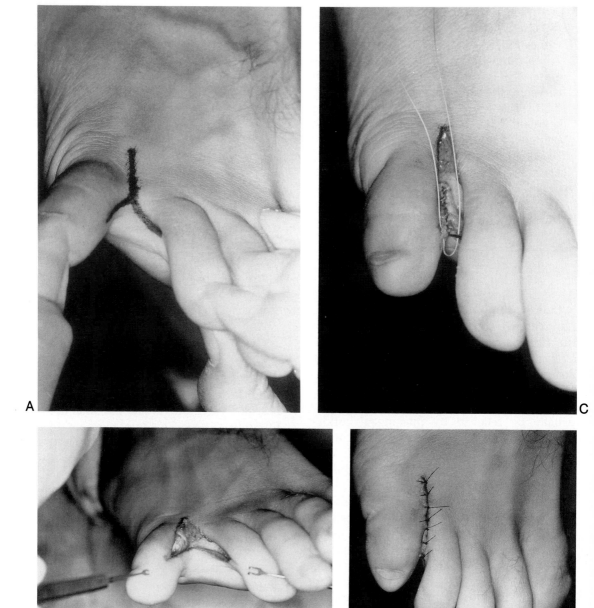

FIGURE 7.8. Syndactylization of toes for a soft corn. (A) Skin is marked for the incision. One distal limb of the Y is drawn; the toes are then pressed together, transferring some of the ink to the adja- cent toe and completing the Y. (B) After excision of the soft corn. (C) Plantar half of the wound is closed with absorbable interrupted stitches. (D) After closure of the dorsal wound.

Postoperative Management. The foot is dressed, and immediate weight-bearing is allowed with a postoperative shoe. The nonabsorbable sutures are removed at 10 to 14 days, and the toes are kept taped together for 2 additional weeks. Full return to activity can proceed when the sutures have been removed.

Metatarsal Head Condylectomy

Technique

1. Under a tourniquet, make a 3 cm S-shaped incision over the MTP and retract laterally or Z-lengthen the extensor tendons, de- pending on the degree of tightness.

2. A dorsal MTP capsulotomy is made longitudinally and the capsule elevated medially and laterally off the head and attachment on the neck of the metatarsal. The joint is plantarflexed 90 degrees, and the entire distal metatarsal cartilage surface is exposed.

3. A small osteotome is used to remove the plantar segment of the metatarsal head and plantar condyle. A rongeur then smooths the remaining bone.

4. The toe is relocated and the capsule closed with interrupted stitches of 3–0 absorbable suture. If the extensor tendons were lengthened, they are repaired with the same suture. The subcutaneous and skin layers are closed separately and a soft dressing applied.

Postoperative Management. Immediate weight-bearing is allowed with a postoperative shoe. The skin sutures are removed at 10 to 14 days, and active and passive range of motion exercises are begun. Walking is allowed in a regular shoe, but running or jumping is delayed for an additional 2 to 4 weeks, depending on the patient's level of discomfort.

Metatarsal Neck Osteotomies

Metatarsal neck osteotomies (Fig. 7.9) are always performed in groups. If the IPK is under the second metatarsal head, the second and third metatarsals are osteotomized. If the IPK is under the fourth metatarsal head, the third and fourth metatarsals are osteotomized. If it is under the third metatarsal head, the second, third, and fourth metatarsals are osteotomized.

Technique

1. Appropriate anesthesia and a tourniquet are used. A 3 cm dorsal longitudinal incision is made beginning distally at the level of the MTP joint. The incision is placed over the third metatarsal for an IPK under the third metatarsal. For an IPK under the second metatarsal head it is placed over the 2–3 intermetatarsal space, and for an IPK under the fourth head metatarsal over the 3–4 intermetatarsal space.

2. Through the appropriate incision, the extensor tendons are retracted and the necks

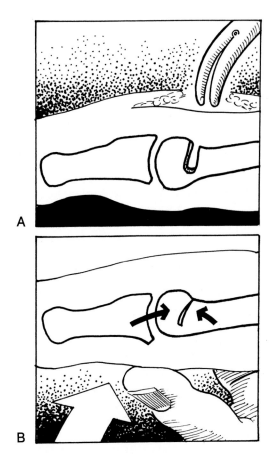

A

B

FIGURE 7.9. Wolf metatarsal neck osteotomy. (A) A small rongeur cuts through the dorsal three-fourths of the metatarsal neck, leaving a plantar hinge intact. (B) With pressure directed upward under the metatarsal head, the plantar hinge cracks, allowing the head to rise.

of the metatarsals to be osteotomized exposed. Use a scalpel to elevate the soft tissue from the medial and lateral sides of the metatarsal neck. A small Hohmann retractor placed along the side of the metatarsal just proximal to the neck aids in visualization.

3. A small rongeur is used to take small bites out of the dorsal neck and then along either side through the cortex of the metatarsal. The dorsal 75% is cut away, leaving an intact plantar hinge. It is important to take multiple small bites because a large bite may crack the bone.

4. Upward pressure is then exerted against the ball of the foot under the metatarsal head, causing the remaining plantar hinge

to crack upward. No fixation is used, and the head finds its own level when walking during the postoperative period.

5. After repeating the osteotomy on the other metatarsal or metatarsals, the wound is closed in layers and dressed.

Postoperative Management. Immediate weight-bearing is allowed in a postoperative shoe. The sutures are removed at 10 to 14 days and use of the postoperative shoe continued for 2 weeks more, at which point regular shoes can be worn. No athletic activities should be attempted for 6 to 8 weeks after surgery.

Sesamoid Intractable Plantar Keratosis

If a fractured sesamoid heals with a distorted shape it may cause an intractable plantar keratosis (IPK) to form (Brodsky, 1993; Leventen, 1991). Increased pressure due to the prominence results in a thick callus that may become painful. Other causes of IPK formation under the first MTP include clawing of the great toe and a cavus foot.

Nonoperative Treatment

The two mainstays of nonoperative treatment are to (1) trim the callus and (2) decrease the pressure under the bony prominence that is responsible for the callus. Intermittent paring with a scalpel can remove large callus buildup but should be done only by a physician. Between these sharp débridements the athlete should regularly scour the callus with an abrasive tool or pumice stone. A pumice works best when the callus has been softened, for instance during the daily bath or shower.

Felt HAPADs or metatarsal pads built into insoles transfer weight-bearing pressure proximally and off the area of the IPK. Cutouts in an orthotic insole under the IPK can further decrease the pressure (Axe and Ray, 1988).

Operative Treatment

The surgical options include complete excision of the abnormal sesamoid or shaving of the plantar one-half to reduce the promi-

nence responsible for callus formation (Brodsky, 1993; Mann and Wapner, 1992).

Sesamoid Shaving

Technique

1. The approach for shaving (Fig. 7.10) is similar to that for excising a sesamoid: The medial sesamoid is approached medially, and the lateral sesamoid is approached through a plantar incision.
2. The joint capsule is exposed, but the joint is not entered. Instead, a longitudinal incision is made in the medial capsule-periosteum of the sesamoid at the midaxial level of the sesamoid. The soft tissue is then subperiosteally elevated from the plantar one-half of the sesamoid with a #15 scalpel.
3. An oscillating saw is used to cut the bone in its middle, parallel to the sole of the foot. The plantar bone is sharply excised, leaving the articular surface intact. Use a small rongeur and rasp to smooth the remaining bone so no sharp edges are prominent.
4. The wound is closed in layers, and a soft dressing is applied.

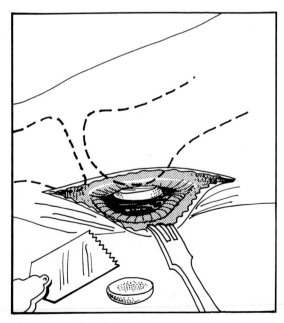

FIGURE 7.10. Sesamoid shaving. Plantar half of the medial sesamoid is removed with an oscillating saw.

Postoperative Management. The patient is kept non-weight-bearing for 10 to 14 days. The skin sutures are then removed, and weight-bearing is allowed in a regular shoe. Athletic activities are resumed after 4 weeks as tolerated.

Plantar Wart

Warts are tumors in the skin caused by the papilloma virus (Glover, 1990; McNerney, 1990). The virus infects the skin, and a cell-mediated immunologic response occurs. The result is the vascular, hyperkeratotic lesion called a wart. Warts may be asymptomatic but, if located on weight-bearing surfaces, can be painful. According to Glover (1990), the peak rates of infection are found in adolescents, and the natural history is for spontaneous resolution with 60% resolving within 2 years.

It is important to differentiate warts from plantar keratoses due to pressure (IPKs) because the treatment for each is different. An IPK is a response to increased pressure with the lesion forming under a bony prominence. Warts may develop in similar locations. Lesions not directly under a pressure area are more likely to be warts. The papillary lines of the skin pass undisturbed through an IPK but are seen to deviate around a wart (Fig. 7.11).

Paring the lesion is part of the treatment of both warts and IPKs and is useful for diagnosis as well. An IPK is formed of hyperkeratotic skin that may have a hard, translucent central core, none of which is vascular. When paring a wart, the superficial layer appears to have multiple dark dots, which are thrombosed arterioles seen end-on. With deeper paring, these vessels begin to bleed, and cessation of bleeding may require pressure applied for several minutes.

Warts may occur as isolated lesions or in multiples. A large wart can be seen with several small satellite warts in close proximity. Multiple small warts may appear to coalesce into a mosaic wart (Fig. 7.12).

Because warts disappear spontaneously over time, treatment is best directed only at those that are symptomatic. There are cosmetic and social issues that accompany warts and can be reasons for their treatment, but they are not good indications for aggressive surgical techniques.

Nonoperative Treatment

HAPADS and orthotic devices can relieve pressure on the wart, resolving the weight-bearing pain. These devices are used in the same manner as for treatment of IPKs. The list of treatments that have been used to eradicate viral warts is protean (Glover, 1990). Good results can be obtained with the use of a topical chemical preparation of lactic and salicylic acid applied on a daily basis by the athlete. This technique has a cure rate of

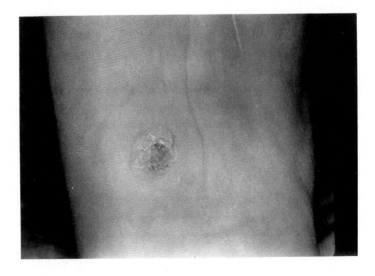

FIGURE 7.11. Solitary plantar wart. Papillary lines of the skin deviate around the lesion. Dark spots indicate end arterioles.

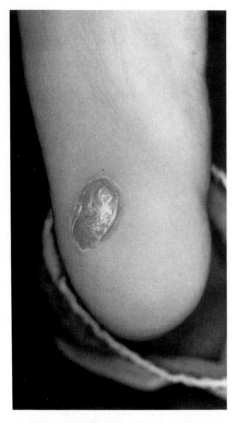

FIGURE 7.12. Large mosaic plantar wart that has resulted after several attempts at surgical excision.

84% in 3 months (Bunney et al., 1976). This simple method allows continued sports participation during treatment. Resistant cases should be referred to a dermatologist for more aggressive treatment.

1. The lesion is first pared by the physician to confirm the diagnosis and remove the hyperkeratotic outer layer. Any bleeding is arrested by direct pressure over the wart for several minutes. The athlete is then instructed in the treatment regimen.
2. The foot is soaked for 5 to 10 minutes in warm water to loosen the overlying cap. The wart is manually débrided by the athlete with a fingernail or small appliance.
3. The topical preparation is placed on the wart and allowed to dry thoroughly. These preparations are mixed with a volatile liquid that evaporates, leaving a firm crust of acid on top of the wart. Weight-bearing

before drying dissipates the preparation. It usually takes 20 to 30 minutes for complete drying, so the athlete is advised to perform this step daily at a time when sitting still is possible. An alternative method is to use a hair dryer, which directs warm air over the applied acid, reducing the drying process to less than 10 minutes.

4. With each ensuing day of treatment, the acid works itself deeper into the base of the wart, which may cause some discomfort for the athlete.
5. The athlete should be examined every 2 to 3 weeks during treatment so regular paring can be done and progress is assessed. It is important to continue the program on a regular daily basis, and it may take 2 to 3 months to eradicate the wart. HAPADS or orthotic insoles can be used at the same time to relieve pressure on the lesion.

Blisters

Blisters are a common problem in athletes whose sport requires quick pivoting and direction changes (Lillich and Baxter, 1986; McNerney, 1990; Sammarco, 1982). Blisters develop when shear forces cause the epidermis to separate from the underlying dermis. A serous exudate fills the space between the layers.

Predisposing causes of blisters include a change in training pattern, shoewear, or training surface, and underlying architectural abnormalities of the foot. Blisters are commonly seen when athletes resume training after a vacation. Shoes that are too narrow or too tight can rub against the skin. Conversely, shoes that are too large may allow the foot to slide within it, causing shear stress on the skin. Running on a synthetic surface with spikes increases friction at the shoe–surface interface, predisposing the foot to slide within the shoe (Lillich and Baxter, 1986). Hammertoes, clawtoes, bunions, and bunionettes are among the deformities that can lead to blistering.

Blisters can be prevented by wearing properly fitting shoes with thick socks. Runners should train on forgiving surfaces that allow some sliding motion between the shoe and surface, thereby decreasing the shear between the foot and shoe (Lillich and Baxter, 1986).

Small blisters are covered with an antibiotic ointment and an adherent padding, such as moleskin. Larger blisters are punctured with a small needle in multiple places to drain the fluid and are then covered with an antibiotic ointment and moleskin (McNerney, 1990).

Athlete's Foot (Tinea Pedis)

Athlete's foot is a fungal infection of the skin that is common in athletes but can occur in all populations. It first manifests as itching and burning in the affected areas, usually between the toes or on the ball of the foot. As it progresses, the skin also becomes dry and scaly. In some athletes blistering occurs, signifying bacterial superinfection (McNerney, 1990).

Diagnosis

The diagnosis is usually made from the history and clinical examinaton. Microscopic examination of a wet mount of skin scrapings in a 10% potassium hydroxide solution reveals branching fungal forms, confirming the diagnosis. A second confirmatory test is to culture tissue scrapings in test tubes on Sabouraud's medium. This technique allows identification of the particular fungus involved. These tests are not practical for all cases of athlete's foot, most of which can be treated based on clinical grounds.

Athlete's foot develops in moist areas of the forefoot. It is particularly common between the toes but may extend onto the plantar or dorsal forefoot. The moist environment promotes the growth of dermatophytes (the fungi) and gram-negative bacteria that also are present on the skin in these areas. The normal acidity of the skin is decreased, which favors the growth of these pathogens.

The fungi initially damage the outer layer of the epidermis, the stratum corneum, which leads to the common dry and scaly athlete's foot, a painful, itchy condition. Bacteria can thrive in the damaged skin, and as they proliferate their release of proteolytic enzymes causes further damage to the skin.

As the action of the fungi and bacteria continue there is an increase in inflammation, and fluid may weep from the affected areas, causing more pain, itching, and redness in the affected areas. At this point bacterial growth may predominate and lead to maceration and erosion of the plantar skin.

Prophylaxis and Treatment

Prevention of athlete's foot is based on good foot hygiene. Clean cotton socks should be worn during athletic activities and changed regularly during prolonged workouts. Immediate showering or bathing after activities with care to clean between the toes prevents the local development of an environment favorable for athlete's foot. Prophylactic application of antifungal powder after cleaning the foot keeps the skin dry and inhibits fungal growth.

Topical antifungal lotion or cream is helpful when the skin becomes dry and scaly, indicating an early case of athlete's foot. Various antifungal agents are available including tolnaftate (Tinactin), miconazole nitrate (Micatin), and clotrimazole (Lotrimin or Mycelex). These medications should be applied twice a day for 2 to 4 weeks. The moisturizer in the cream helps prevent fissures from forming in the skin, which can lead to bacterial superinfection. Treatment should be continued for the full duration even after the infection seems to have resolved.

If there is weeping of fluid or blistering, soaks should be performed two or three times daily for 10 minutes with tap water and soap. At this stage bacterial infection has occurred, and oral antibiotics should be administered. Potassium permanganate can be painted onto the skin. When the foot has stabilized, topical antifungal cream or lotion is applied. Oral antifungal agents should be avoided when treating athlete's foot, as they have significant side effects that include headaches, gastrointestinal upset and rarely hepatitis. If there is no improvement with topical antifungal treatment, a dermatologic evaluation should be obtained.

Toenail Disorders

Toenail problems include fungal infection, overgrowth, ingrowth, and infection. These common disorders occur in all populations and can seriously affect athletic performance.

Anatomy

The toenail is a specialized unit composed of five parts: the nail plate, nail bed, nail matrix, hyponychium, and nail folds (Fig. 7.13) (Dixon, 1983; Eisele, 1994; Fleckman, 1985). The nail plate is a tissue made of several layers of keratinized cells that grow out of the germinal nail matrix and rest on the nail bed. It has a low water content and a high sulfur content, which contribute to its hardness (Coughlin, 1993). The stiffness of the nail plate provides rigidity for the soft tissue at the distal ends of the toes.

The toenail matrix extends medially and laterally the entire width of the nail and proximally about 5 mm from the cuticle, where the skin laps down on the nail plate. The lunula, seen under the proximal nail plate as a light-colored crescent, is the distal extent of the matrix. It then becomes continuous with the nail bed. The matrix contains basal cells that form the nail plate.

The nail bed is an epithelial surface with longitudinal grooves that supports the nail plate (Fleckman, 1985). The undersurface of the plate and the grooves in the bed form a strong bond that holds them firmly together.

The distal end of this attachment is called the hyponychium.

Along the medial and lateral borders of the nail lie the nail folds. They are the curved areas of skin that abut the nail plate. There is also a proximal nail fold where the dorsal skin of the toe meets the nail plate at the cuticle. The deep surface of the proximal nail fold is called the eponychium and is firmly attached to the plate (Dixon, 1983; Fleckman, 1985).

The nail grows distally about 1 mm each month. The normal shape of the toenail complex causes growth to occur in this direction. Injury to the toenail can cause upward instead of distal growth or growth against the nail folds, leading to a distorted or ingrown toenail (Coughlin, 1993).

Clinical Presentation

Any of the components of the toenail complex can be involved in disease or become injured. Common problems are seen in the nail plate, nail bed, and medial and lateral nail folds. Disorders of the nail plates generally cause the nail to thicken. Nails that have become thick or overgrown can irritate the nail folds, leading to painful ingrowing. They may also rub against the skin of an adjacent toe, causing pain and irritation. Thickening is due to a variety of causes including fungal and bacterial infection, congenital deformity, systemic disease, trauma, and aging.

Eradication of fungal infection in a toenail

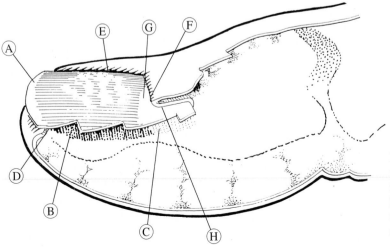

FIGURE 7.13. Nail complex. A, nail plate; B, nail bed; C, nail matrix; D, hyponichium; E, lateral nail fold; F, proximal nail fold; G, lunula; H, eponychium.

is virtually impossible unless the nail plate is removed. Topical antifungals do not diffuse adequately through the nail plate to eliminate the infection. Because these infections rarely cause symptoms, the best treatment is to keep the shape of the nail as normal as possible with regular trimming and thinning with a burr as needed to prevent mechanical problems. In severe cases the nail plate is removed and topical antifungal medication applied to the underlying base.

Nails can become ingrown and lead to pain or infection at the nail margin, a condition that most commonly involves the great toenail. The nail should be cut straight across, which allows it to grow out unimpeded. Nails that are cut at an angle may have an edge that digs into the marginal skin, causing pressure and ingrowth. A torn nail, thickened nail, or congenitally incurving nail may also develop this problem. Shoes or socks that are tight can put pressure against the edge of the nail (Fig. 7.14).

Any of these factors may lead to a localized area of ischemia in the nail margin that is painful and inflamed, the first stage of ingrowth (Heifitz, 1961). Infection with edema and drainage mark the second stage of ingrowing. Finally, granulation tissue forms with chronic infection, and the lateral wall hypertrophies (Fig. 7.15).

Nail bed disorders are generally caused by trauma. Laceration of the nail bed can lead to

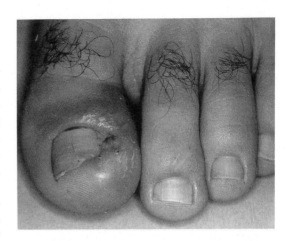

FIGURE 7.15. Ingrown toenail. Chronic infection is present with granulation tissue and hypertrophy of the lateral wall.

chronic distortion of the overlying nail plate. The laceration may communicate with the underlying phalanx, and a radiograph should be obtained to ensure that an open fracture has not occurred (Mortimer and Dawber, 1985). If a laceration is present, the bed should be repaired after removal of the nail plate. If the plate can be salvaged, it can be placed over the top of the repaired nail bed to act as a splint. Appropriate antibiotic therapy is provided to cover against *Staphylococcus aureus*, the most common pathogen (Eisele, 1994).

A subungual hematoma is due to bleeding that occurs from the nail bed into the space between the bed and plate. It can be caused by a direct blow, such as dropping an object on the end of the toe or if someone steps on the toe. Trauma due to the end of the toe striking a toebox that is too tight may also lead to a subungual hematoma (Fig. 7.16). This situation sometimes occurs with downhill running, which tends to force the toe against the front of the shoe. Increased pressure caused by the hemorrhage is painful but can be easily relieved by drilling with a red-hot needle.

Treatment

Prevention is the best form of treatment. Shoes should have an adequate toebox, and socks must fit well. It is important to cut the

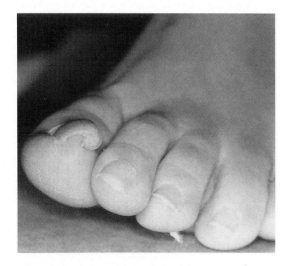

FIGURE 7.14. Incurving nail. The great toenail is curved under, making trimming difficult.

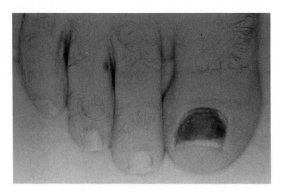

Figure 7.16. Subungual hematoma. Running in shoes that are too tight can lead to bleeding under the great toenail.

nails regularly and straight across, not obliquely at the edges. For nails that are deformed or thickened, clippers may not be adequate, and a small hand burr may be necessary to thin the nail first. Care should be taken when using a burr not to let it slip off and burn the skin. Moreover, the burr can generate significant heat, so it must be used slowly when working on thick nails.

An acute subungual hematoma can cause significant pain due to pressure under the nail. Such pain is relieved by drilling a hole through the nail to allow the fluid to escape.

The nail plate is removed from fungus-infected nails or nails that are congenitally deformed or have been damaged by trauma. The nail is removed and a new nail allowed to grow back in its place.

An ingrown nail that is painful but does not have erythema in the marginal tissue can be treated with soaks twice a day and by placing a small piece of cotton gauze under the distal edge of the nail (Bordelon, 1985; Eisele, 1994). This treatment may relieve the pressure against the nail margin and prevent local ischemia. If the nail margin is erythematous, an oral antibiotic can be added to this regimen for several days (Eisele, 1994). Should the problem not resolve or even worsen, or if purulence is present, the nail margin is removed. If it is a recurrent problem, a chemical matrixectomy is performed. The Heifitz procedure—surgical excision of the nail edge and marginal skin—is used for failures of chemical matrixectomy (Pettine et al., 1988).

Subungual Hematoma Drainage

1. A digital block is provided with lidocaine, and the toe is prepared with an antiseptic solution. An 18 gauge needle is placed on a syringe to act as a handle. The tip of the needle is heated with a match until it glows red. It is then used to drill down through the nail plate over the hematoma in one or more spots to release the fluid.
2. The toe is dressed and the dressing removed the next day for soaking in tap water and soap. There should be immediate relief of pain with release of pressure. Activities can be safely advanced as the symptoms allow.

Nail Plate Avulsion

1. A digital block is performed with lidocaine, and the toe is prepared with an antiseptic solution. A penrose drain can be used as a tourniquet at the base of the toe but is not usually needed.
2. A Freer elevator or other blunt tool is passed under the nail plate and is worked back and forth, pressing proximally to the matrix. The instrument is then run between the nail plate and the cuticle to free it dorsally. The nail is grasped with a hemostat and pulled free.
3. A small piece of petrolatum gauze is placed over the nail bed and worked under the cuticle. It is covered with a cotton 2 × 2 gauze and held in place with a toe wrap. The dressing is removed after 24 hours and the toe is gently washed during daily bathing. Athletic activities can be resumed within 1 to 2 days.
4. When treating a fungal infection, topical antifungal cream is rubbed into the nail bed daily. When the tenderness resolves, after 3 to 5 days, the athlete is instructed to use a soft bristle toothbrush to gently débride the nail bed during bathing or showering prior to applying the antifungal cream. This regimen should be undertaken daily until the nail has regrown.

Nail Margin Excision

1. A digital block is performed with lidocaine, and the toe is prepared with an

antiseptic solution. A Penrose drain can be used as a tourniquet at the base of the toe but is not usually needed.

2. One tip of a small scissors is placed under the nail 2 mm from the margin on the ingrown side. The scissors are then used to cut proximally along the entire edge. At the proximal end the upper tip is forced under the cuticle so the nail is cut but the cuticle is left intact.

3. A Freer elevator is passed around the cut segment bluntly, freeing it from the soft tissue. It is grasped with a hemostat and avulsed.

4. The edge is then packed with a petrolatum gauze and covered with a cotton 2 × 2 gauze and toe wrap.

5. The dressing is removed after 24 hours, and the toe is soaked twice a day in soapy water for 5 to 10 minutes. A bandaid and an open-toe or loose-fitting shoe are worn for a few days until the patient is symptom-free. Athletic activities can be resumed at that point.

Chemical Matrixectomy

1. Chemical matrixectomy (Fig 7.17) is performed exactly like a nail margin excision. When the nail segment has been removed, phenol (carbolic acid) is placed into the depth of the proximal wound to chemically ablate the nail matrix.

2. The skin at the base of the toe is first covered with petrolatum gauze to protect it. A cotton tip applicator is then dipped into phenol and placed against the matrix for 5 seconds, twirling it in the depths of the wound. This step is repeated three times.

3. The wound is then copiously flushed with alcohol and the skin cleansed to ensure that no phenol remains, which can cause a chemical burn.

4. The wound is then packed with a petrolatum gauze and covered with a cotton 2 × 2 gauze and a toe wrap. The dressing is removed after 24 hours and the toe soaked twice a day in soapy water for 5 to 10 minutes. There may be weeping fluid from the base of the wound for up to 2 weeks, so the toe should be covered with a band-aid until it stops. An open-toed or loose-fitting shoe is worn until the patient is symptom-free. Athletic activities can be resumed at that point.

Heifitz Procedure

The Heifitz procedure (Fig. 7.18) should be performed at a surgery center rather than in an office setting.

1. A digital block is performed with lidocaine, and a Penrose drain is used as a tourniquet at the base of the toe. Alternatively, an ankle block with a Esmarch ankle tourniquet or general anesthesia with a thigh tourniquet can be used.

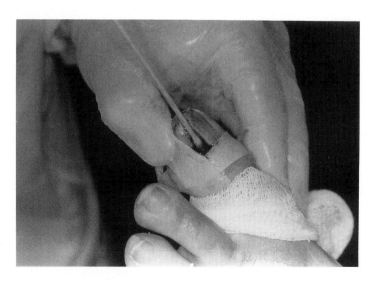

FIGURE 7.17. Chemical matrixectomy. After excision of the lateral nail edge, phenol is applied to the matrix with a cotton-tipped applicator.

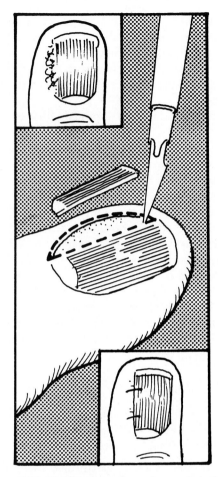

FIGURE 7.18. Heifitz procedure for a chronic ingrown toenail. (A) Nail with granulation tissue along the edge. (B) Nail edge and lateral nail fold are excised, removing the granulation tissue. (C) Edge of the skin is closed against the edge of the nail with simple stitches.

2. A #15 scalpel is used to make a longitudinal incision parallel to the nail edge 2 mm from the marginal skin. The incision runs from the distal level of the nail to a point 2 mm proximal to it, to where the nail fold curves. It then turns to the base of the nail. Any granulation tissue due to chronic infection is included. The incision should continue hard to bone.
3. Scissors with sharp tips are passed under the nail plate 2 mm from the edge, and the nail is split longitudinally. A Freer elevator then separates this segment from the rest of the nail, and the segment is removed with the excised skin margin.

4. A wedge of matrix is then sharply removed using the scalpel. The base is finally débrided with a curet to ensure that no small pieces of matrix are left behind that could give rise to a spicule of nail.
5. The skin is then closed against the nail. Three simple stitches of 3–0 nonabsorbable suture are passed through the skin and the new nail edge, drawing the skin against the nail.
6. The toe is covered with a cotton 2 × 2 gauze and a toe wrap. Immediate weight-bearing is allowed with a postoperative shoe. The sutures are removed at 10 to 14, days and shoewear is advanced. Athletic activities can be resumed after 4 weeks.

Foreign Bodies and Puncture Wounds

The foot is a common site of puncture wounds and penetrating injuries that introduce foreign bodies. These injuries occur most often when barefoot, but some puncture injuries do occur through the sole of the shoe (Jacobs et al., 1982). Most of these injuries are caused by wood or glass splinters and are superficial, being satisfactorily treated by the athlete with home instruments such as tweezers and sewing needles. Deeper injuries may be caused by wood splinters and glass, as well as toothpicks, needles, and nails (Cracchiolo, 1980; Rimoldi and Gogan, 1991). These deeper injuries occur most commonly in the ball of the foot and the heel and less often under the arch.

Clinical Presentation

Puncture wounds in the foot are painful and most often immediately recognized. If a piece of foreign material is retained in the foot, it can cause immediate or delayed pain (Markiewitz et al., 1994). Migration of foreign bodies that were initially insignificant to the patient can produce new symptoms. On occasion, an asymptomatic foreign body is identified on a radiograph obtained for an unrelated injury or condition. These injuries can safely be neglected, to be dealt with only if symptoms subsequently develop (Alfred and Jacobs, 1984).

Infection is the most feared consequence of a puncture wound. Organisms can be inoculated by objects first penetrating the shoe prior to entering the skin (Jacobs et al., 1982). The most common organism involved in puncture infections is *Staphylococcus aureus* (Sammarco, 1993). *Pseudomonas aeruginosa* and other gram-negative bacteria are found in injuries where the sole of the shoe was first penetrated (Rimoldi and Gogan, 1991). Toothpicks may be associated with bacteria from the oral cavity and cause anaerobic infections. The athlete's tetanus status must be ascertained and appropriate treatment provided.

Radiography

Radiographs should be obtained, although many objects, including wood and most types of glass, cannot be visualized (Fig. 7.19). Xeroradiography has been used but has limitations in terms of its ability to identify wooden foreign bodies (Anderson et al., 1982). Magnetic resonance imaging (MRI) and ultrasonography can be used to identify radiolucent objects. The use of a portable ultrasonography machine by an emergency room physician with only basic experience has been shown to be a sensitive test for identifying these nonopaque foreign bodies (Schlager et al., 1991). Both MRI and ultrasonography are better at detecting foreign objects if they are not in close proximity to bone (Mizel et al., 1994).

Treatment

If the object has been identified, it should be removed as soon as possible. Treatment is often attempted in the emergency department, where the conditions are suboptimal. The operating room or outpatient surgery center is preferable because of better light, instruments, and assistance. An ankle block anesthetic or general anesthesia should be given to allow satisfactory exploration of the wound. Triangulation using needles placed on the skin and visualization using an image intensifier (fluoroscopy) can help to localize radiopaque objects intraoperatively.

The wound is packed open and allowed to close secondarily. Non-weight-bearing with crutches expedites wound healing without irritation. The original dressing is removed after 2 to 3 days, and subsequent dressings are changed daily. Development of infection requires antibiotics based on culture and sensitivity reports. Return to training is allowed when the skin has healed.

Thermal Injuries

Thermal injuries are due to exposure to extremes of high or low temperature. Burns occur much more commonly than cold inju-

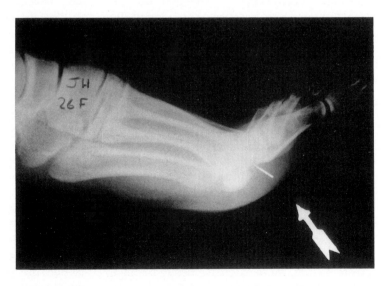

FIGURE 7.19. Foreign body in the foot. Broken piece of a needle is seen under the forefoot on a plain radiograph.

ries in the general population. Burns are uncommon among athletes, occurring when the foot comes in contact with a hot object: a liquid spill on the foot or when a heating pad is left against the foot for an extended time. Cold injuries are found in some groups of athletes because of the environment in which they play. Winter sports such as alpine and cross-country skiing, outdoor skating, snowmobile racing, and mountain climbing often expose the participant to the dangers of a cold injury.

Burns of the Foot

The athlete's foot is usually protected from burn injury by shoewear. Most burns occur not during training but, rather, during a domestic accident. They usually result from spilling hot liquid on the top of the foot or brushing against a hot object such as an iron or radiator. An electrical burn may result from contact with a live wire, causing current to pass through the foot. A chemical burn is due to contact with an acid or base that causes a direct chemical reaction with the tissue; it can generate significant heat as it reacts (Sammarco, 1993; Stanitski, 1985).

Clinical Presentation

Burns initially appear erythematous and blanch with pressure. After 24 hours, areas that have been severely damaged do not blanch on pressure because of damage to the capillary bed. These areas become white and may undergo necrosis. Burns are classified by the extent of tissue damage as first, second, or third degree injuries (Sammarco, 1993).

A first degree burn is superficial and is characterized by erythema without blistering. A second degree burn is also superficial, with erythema accompanied by blistering. This partial-thickness injury to the skin involves damage that extends through the epidermis to involve a portion of the dermis. A third degree burn damages the full thickness of the skin, both epidermis and dermis, and may extend to the deeper muscle, connective tissue and bone. Electrical burns generally create deeper, more extensive tissue damage than is initially apparent.

Treatment

The margins of a burn may remain overheated when the causative agent is removed, causing extension of injury. Therefore it is important to cool the area as soon as possible. The foot can be immersed in a cool water bath or placed under cool running water. Blisters should be left intact and the skin covered with an antiseptic petroleum jelly gauze. Second and third degree burns usually require hospitalization for treatment that may include intravenous fluid replacement, antibiotics, regular dressing changes, débridement, and skin grafting (Deitch, 1990).

With electrical burns the foot should be dressed and splinted and the patient hospitalized for further treatment. Radiographs should be obtained to determine if any bone damage has occurred. Treatment is then similar to that for third-degree thermal burns.

Chemical burns should be treated by copious irrigation of the skin with running water to dilute and wash off the irritant. Extensive chemical burns should be dressed and splinted, followed by in-hospital treatment (Sammarco, 1993).

Cold Injuries of the Foot

When considering the effects of cold on the body, it is useful to differentiate the core from the extremities. The core consists of the brain, heart, lungs, and abdominal organs; and the extremities are primarily muscle, skin, and bones. The human body generates heat through the oxidation of metabolic constituents. In the resting state this reaction occurs at a constant rate and is termed basal heat production. The body functions properly with temperature regulated between a few degrees of 37° C (Fritz and Perrin, 1989; Grace, 1987).

The extremities are involved in thermoregulation. The blood supply of the extremities works as a heat exchanger. Vessels are arranged to shunt warm arterial blood from the depths of the extremity to the superficial veins, where heat is transferred to the tissues and then the environment.

When the body becomes cold, there are several mechanisms for increasing heat production. Shivering is caused by muscular action and can increase heat production three to four times the basal rate. Purposeful muscular activity produces heat at different rates, depending on the intensity of the activity. Mild or moderate intensity activity can produce heat nearly five times the basal rate and can usually be maintained for an extended time. High intensity activity may produce heat approaching 10 times basal activity but can be maintained for only brief periods (Sammarco, 1993).

In addition to generating more heat, the thermoregulatory mechanisms in the extremities are activated when the temperature drops. Shunting of blood to the skin is rapidly halted.

Pathogenesis

Cold injury occurs in two general ways. The first is when the core temperature is maintained, but there is local injury to the extremities. This situation can lead to frostnip, chilblains, trench foot, superficial frostbite, and deep frostbite. The second type of injury occurs when the core temperature falls as does the temperature in the extremities. This situation can cause deep frostbite locally; the drop in core temperature leads to hypothermia, which can progress to death (Grace, 1987).

There are certain factors that predispose to cold injuries. Fatigue limits the ability to generate heat. Alcohol use increases the shunting of blood to the superficial veins in the extremities, initially causing warmth but hastening the body's loss of heat and the drop in core temperature. Constrictive clothing, especially footwear, decreases circulation in the lower extremity. Inadequate insulation from cold and especially the wind causes heat loss. Wet clothing or immersion in cold water leads to a rapid loss of heat, resulting in cold injury (Fritz and Perrin, 1989; Sammarco, 1993).

Frostnip (First Degree Frostbite)

Frostnip, or first degree frostbite, is a superficial injury to the skin of the extremities or face that occurs in extreme cold or high wind conditions and leads to partial freezing of the skin (AAOS, 1991; Delano et al., 1991; Grace, 1987). It may occur quickly and painlessly, with the athlete unaware. It appears as a blanching of the skin and can be treated with application of a warm hand or blowing warm air over the area in the field. With warming there may be tingling in the tissue, but no permanent damage occurs.

Second Degree Frostbite

The next stage is second degree, or superficial, frostbite (AAOS, 1991; Delano et al., 1991). Freezing involves the full thickness of skin. The skin is white and feels firm, although the deeper tissue is soft. With thawing, the tissue becomes edematous and ecchymotic due to damage to blood vessels. Deeper damage may appear as blistering and eschar formation. The area initially is numb with a subsequent burning sensation that can last for weeks. The area is extremely sensitive to reexposure to cold.

Treatment involves rewarming, being careful not to rub or further irritate the tissues. The foot is immersed in a bath of warm (40°–42° C) water, keeping the foot off the sides of the container in order to maintain uniform heating of the foot. The temperature should be regularly checked by thermometer and warm water added as the bath cools. The rewarming continues until the tissue becomes reddened.

At the same time the foot is being treated, the athlete's core temperature must be maintained or raised. Cold and wet clothing is removed and replaced with warm, loose-fitting garb. Warm, nonalcoholic drinks are administered. Analgesic medication may be needed to treat pain, which manifests during rewarming.

Deep Frostbite

Deep frostbite describes freezing of the skin and subcutaneous tissue and can involve the underlying muscle, connective tissue, and bone (Delano et al., 1991; Grace, 1987; Sammarco, 1993). The skin is white and cold, feeling frozen solid to touch.

Hospitalization as soon as possible is necessary, but rewarming treatment as for superficial frostbite is instituted immediately. If there is hypothermia, the core temperature is

treated first, with extremity rewarming subsequently. As thawing occurs, the injured
area appears purple or black. This event is
painful, requiring analgesics. Large blisters
form, and gangrene may be evident within 1
to 2 days.

After rewarming, the foot is carefully ban-
daged, with cotton pads placed between the
toes. Sterile techniques should be used because of the risk of infection in the damaged
skin. Blisters are left intact.

A posterior splint maintains the foot and
ankle in the neutral position. The splint is
removed on several occasions during the day
for range-of-motion exercises. Daily whirlpool treatments at 38° C followed by air-
drying and reapplication of sterile dressings
are used to clean the foot.

In the event of infection, early débridement is performed. Without infection, débridement can be deferred for 2 to 3 weeks, when
demarcation is apparent.

Trench Foot

Trench foot develops when the foot has been
exposed to cold water for an extended time
(Sammarco, 1993). It is characterized by
damage to the capillary circulation in the skin
and progresses to involve the muscle and
nerves.

The foot is initially cold, waxy, and mottled,
with the patient complaining of numbness. As
rewarming occurs, the foot becomes swollen
and red secondary to hyperemia. Blisters may
form, and areas that were significantly damaged appear cyanotic or gangrenous.

The foot is immediately removed from the
cold, wet footwear and is rewarmed in a
water bath between 40°–42° C, as for frostbite. Hospitalization is recommended. Antibiotic therapy and regular dressing changes
under sterile conditions prevent superinfection of the damaged tissue. Débridement and
amputation of gangrenous areas should be
delayed for several weeks until demarcation
has occurred.

Chilblain

Chilbain occurs when an area has been repeatedly exposed to low temperatures for

prolonged periods (AAOS, 1991). The usual
area of foot involvement is the dorsum of
the toes. The exposure causes a chronic inflammatory reaction in the vasculature of
the skin and subcutaneous tissue. Microscopic evaluation of chilblain reveals evidence of perivascular infiltration and intimal
proliferation.

The injured area appears red and swollen,
and it may be hot, tender, and pruritic.
Repeated exposure to cold causes this appearance; and unless it is well established, it
reverts to normal appearance when the cold
has been removed.

The treatment is avoidance of the cold. The
athlete is advised to abandon tight-fitting
shoes and socks in favor of well insulated and
loose-fitting shoewear.

References

Alfred RH, Jacobs R: Occult foreign bodies of the
foot. Foot Ankle 4:209–211, 1984

American Academy of Orthopaedic Surgeons: Environmental problems. In: American Academy
of Orthopaedic Surgeons, Athletic Training
and Sports Medicine, 2nd ed, pp 849–867,
Rosemont, IL, AAOS, 1991

American Academy of Orthopaedic Surgeons: The
skin. In American Academy of Orthopaedic
Surgeons, Athletic Training and Sports Medicine, 2nd ed, pp 441–452, Rosemont, IL,
AAOS, 1991

Anderson MA, Newmeyer WL, Kilgore ES: Diagnosis and treatment of retained foreign bodies
in the hand. Am J Surg 144:63–67, 1982

Axe MJ, Ray RL: Orthotic treatment of sesamoid
pain. Am J Sports Med 16:411–416, 1988

Bordelon RL: Management of disorders of the
forefoot and toenails associated with running.
Clin Sports Med 4:717–724, 1985

Brodsky JW: Disorders of the great oe sesamoids.
In: Myerson M (ed): Current Therapy in Foot
and Ankle Surgery. pp 7–12. St. Louis, Mosby-
Year Book, 1993

Bunney MH, Nolan MW, Williams DA: An assessment of methods of treating viral warts by
comparative treatment trials based on a standard design. Br J Dermatol 89:667–679, 1976

Coughlin MJ: Toenail Abnormalities. In, Mann,
RA and Coughlin, MJ (ed). Surgery of the Foot
and Ankle, pp 1033–1071, St. Louis, Mosby,
1993

Cracchiolo A: Office practice: footwear and orthotic therapy.Foot Ankle 2:242–248, 1982

Cracchiolo A: Wooden foreign bodies in the foot. Am J Surg 140:585–587, 1980

Deitch EA: The management of burns. N Engl J Med 323:1249–1253, 1990

Delano DL, Dascombe WH, Rodriguez A: New horizons in management of hypothermia and frostbite injury. Contemp Probl Trauma Surg 71:345–370, 1991

Dixon GL: Treatment of ingrown toenail. Foot Ankle 3:254–260, 1983

Eisele SA: Conditions of the toenails. Orthop Clin North Am 25:183–188, 1994

Fleckman P: Anatomy and physiology of the nail. Dermatol Clin 3:373–381, 1985

Fritz RL, Perrin DH: cold exposure injuries: prevention and treatment. Clin Sports Med 8:111–126, 1989

Glover MG: Plantar warts. Foot Ankle 11:172–178, 1990

Grace TG: Cold exposure injuries and the winter athlete. Clin Orthop 216:55–62, 1987

Hayda R, Tremaine MD, Tremaine K, et al: Effect of metatarsal pads and their positioning: a quantitative assessment. Foot Ankle 15:561–566, 1994

Heifitz CJ: Ingrown toe-nail: a clinical study. Am J Surg 38:298–315, 1961

Holmes GB, Timmerman L: A quantitative assessment of the effect of metatarsal pads on plantar pressures. Foot Ankle 11:141–145, 1990

Jacobs RF, Adelman L, Sack CM, Wilson CB: Management of Pseudomonas osteochondritis complicating puncture wounds of the foot. Pediatrics 69:432–435, 1982

Jahss MH, Michelson JD, Desai P, et al: Investigations into the fat pads of the sole of the foot: anatomy and histology. Foot Ankle 13:233–242, 1992

Leventen EO: Sesamoid disorders and treatment: an update. Clin Orthop 269:236–240, 1991

Leventen EO, Pearson SW: Distal metatarsal osteotomy for intractable plantar keratoses. Foot Ankle 10:247–251, 1990

Lillich JS, Baxter DE: Common forefoot problems in runners. Foot Ankle 7:145–151, 1986

Mann RA, Wapner K: Tibial sesamoid shaving for treatment of intractable plantar keratosis under the tibial sesamoid. Foot Ankle 13:196–198, 1992

Markiewitz AD, Karns DJ, Brooks PJ: Late infection of the foot due to incomplete removal of foreign bodies: a report of two cases. Foot Ankle 15:52–55, 1994

McNerney JE: Sports-medicine considerations of lesser metatarsalgia. Clin Podiatr Med Surg 7:645–665, 1990

Mizel MS, Steinmetz ND, Trepman E: Detection of wooden foreign bodies in muscle tissue: experimental comparison of computed tomography, magnetic resonance imaging, and untrasonography. Foot Ankle 15:437–443, 1994

Mortimer PS, Dawber RPR: Trauma to the nail unit including occupational sports injuries. Dermatol Clin 3:415–420, 1985

Pettine KA, Cofield RH, Johnson KA, Bussey RM: Ingrown toenail: results of surgical treatment. Foot Ankle 9:130–134, 1988

Rimoldi RL, Gogan WJ: Pseudomonal osteomyelitis of the medial sesamoid bone. South Med J 84:800–801, 1991

Robbins S, Gouw GJ, McClaran J, Waked E: Protective sensation of the plantar aspect of the foot. Foot Ankle 14:347–352, 1993

Sammarco GJ: Miscellaneous soft-tissue injuries. In: Mann RA, Coughlin MJ (eds): Surgery of the Foot and Ankle, pp 1411–1438. St. Louis, Mosby, 1993

Sammarco GJ: Soft tissue conditions in athletes feet. Clin Sports Med 1:149–155, 1982

Schlager D, Sanders AB, Wiggins D, Boren W: Ultrasound for the detection of foreign bodies. Ann Emerg Med 20:189–191, 1991

Sclamberg EL, Lorenz MA: A dorsal wedge V osteotomy for painful plantar callosities. Foot Ankle 4:30–32, 1983

Stanitski CL: Environmental problems of runners. Clin Sports Med 4:725–733, 1985

Wolf MD: Metatarsal osteotomy for the relief of painful metatarsal callosities. J Bone Joint Surg Am 55:1760–1762, 1973

8
Orthotics, Bracing, and Taping

The Role of Athletic Footwear

Athletic shoewear has two basic functions. The first, fundamental requirement is that it must protect the foot. The second is to act as an interface between the body and the functional surface. Highly specialized footwear has developed for most sports that provides these two functions. Consider the contrast between a ski boot and a ballerina's slipper, each of which has evolved to optimize athletic performance.

The shoe can protect the foot from multiple forces. Impact stresses from running and jumping are increased multifold over normal weight-bearing activity. Cushioning in the sole of the shoe dampens the ground reaction force and dissipates this energy, relieving loading of the foot. Improved cushioning has been shown to decrease the incidence of metatarsal and calcaneal stress fractures in runners (Cook et al., 1985). Significant torque may be generated in the foot during athletics (Andreasson et al., 1986). A football player must be able to change direction quickly after foot-plant and cannot tolerate shoe slippage on the playing surface. The cleats on the shoe prevent it from slipping when torque is applied. If the traction is too great, however, there is an increased risk for sustaining rotational injuries of the ankle or knee (Torg, 1982). Similarly, tennis players on clay surfaces must be able to quickly change directions, which requires good traction. The

same shoe, however, must allow them to slide on the clay in controlled fashion when extending to reach a ball hit to the far side of the court. Shoes must also protect players whose feet must undergo rapid acceleration and deceleration, often in many planes. A basketball player, for example, is involved in running with quick stops and starts, lateral movements, and jumping and landing motions.

Shoewear also protects the foot from the environment. Extremes of temperature that would not be tolerated by the foot alone can be tolerated with the proper shoe. A long distance runner can compete on an asphalt surface on a hot summer day, and a cross-country skier can compete in the coldest winter conditions. The shoe also protects the foot against damage due to irregularities in the surface, which allows running cross-country through rock, gravel, and other hazards.

The second main function of shoewear is to act as an interface between the playing surface and the foot. To perform, there must be efficient transfer of energy from the athlete by way of the foot to the athletic surface. Additionally, there is a transfer of information about the surface back through the shoe to the athlete ("feel"). A shoe that is too loose or poorly constructed may not efficiently transfer energy from the foot to the surface. This situation may be seen in the extreme with alpine ski boots. Here the torque applied by the leg and foot through the boot is efficiently transferred to the edge of the ski, causing it to turn. A boot that is too soft may be more comfortable but does not turn the ski as efficiently.

Cushioning and support are important, and flexibility is yet another factor. If a shoe is too stiff, it can irritate the skin and may not allow the necessary foot and ankle motions needed to perform the sport. The ballerina's slipper provides important support in the forefoot while allowing full and unrestricted motion in the midfoot, hindfoot, and ankle.

Another important factor is that the shoe transmits sensory information back to the body. The athlete is unconsciously feeling the environment, the surface, through the interface of the shoe, which for instance allows a basketball player to feel a slippery spot on the floor. A skier can tell the texture of the snow and instantly knows if there is hard ice or a soft spot, allowing the body to correct for the difference. The ability to make instantaneous corrections for the position of the foot enables the runner to maintain balance on an irregular surface based on proprioceptive information received through the shoe. If the shoe is poorly designed and does not allow for this feel, the athlete's performance may be hampered.

Advances in material sciences have made dramatic changes in athletic shoewear in recent years (Torg, 1982). Until recently all shoes were leather or canvas. The development of plastic injection techniques and closed and open cell foams have provided many specialized materials that can be fashioned together to make shoes for a specific function.

The most important factor about athletic shoewear, no matter what sport is involved, is the fit of the shoe (Mann, 1993; Torg, 1982). Shoes that are loose not only decrease the positive feel the athlete needs for the surface, they can cause increased shear forces on the skin, which can lead to blisters and nail problems from jamming against the end of the toebox. Conversely, shoes that are too tight may cause callus formation and over the long term can cause a multitude of deformities in the toes including hallux valgus, bun-ions, hammertoes, and bunionettes. The importance of careful fitting of athletic shoewear cannot be overstated.

Shoe Modifications

A variety of modifications can be made directly to the shoe to improve or maintain function when foot pathology is encountered. These modifications differ from orthotics, which are devices placed in the shoe (Janisse, 1994).

An extra-depth shoe can be used to accommodate an orthotic insert. It may also help the athlete with claw toes or hammertoes that are being rubbed by a conventional shoe. Most running shoes are made with removable insoles, and simply replacing them with a thinner insole may provide the extra depth needed to accommodate these deformities.

Athletes with bunions or bunionettes may experience pain from pressure against the deformity. Obtaining a shoe that is wider in the forefoot is not always possible, as it then may be too loose in the hindfoot. The pressure areas can be relieved by stretching the shoe over the areas of the deformity or sewing a balloon patch over it.

A rocker-bottom sole is built to allow for rolling of the foot from heel-strike to toe-off without the shoe significantly flexing. This modification is used when there is stiffness in the foot that does not allow normal motion. It can be used for hallux rigidus or after midfoot or ankle trauma that results in stiffness. The sole is usually stiffened with a fiberglass or spring steel shank built into the sole.

A solid ankle cushion heel (SACH) is a wedge of shock-absorbing cushion added to the sole in the heel. It is often added to the rocker-bottom sole construct. It can be used by itself to improve cushioning in athletes with chronic heel pain.

A flare is an extension along the medial or lateral side of the sole that provides stability to the foot. A lateral flare can be used in athletes with a cavus foot or those with a tendency to roll laterally off the side of their foot, sustaining inversion injuries.

Orthoses

An orthosis is a device that fits into a shoe to improve function. Various types of orthoses exist. The major effects of orthoses are to increase cushioning, maintain alignment, and alter the weight-bearing stresses in specific areas of the foot. Given the continual striving by athletes, coaches, and trainers to enhance performance, orthoses are widely used. Unfortunately, much of what is attributed to orthoses has not been confirmed by scientific studies.

Canting of ski boots enjoyed great popularity during the 1970s as a means of improving edge control of the ski. The sole of the ski boot was posted either medially or laterally based on the position of the skier's leg when standing on a swiveling base while wearing the boot. In fact, this modification is unncessary except in extreme cases of lower extremity malalignment.

Longitudinal orthoses have been used widely by runners to treat excessive pronation of the foot, which is often regarded as the universal cause of any malady. The use of orthotic devices with a medial support can decrease the amount and rate of pronation when tested in the laboratory (Lutter, 1980; Mann et al., 1981); however, they also increase the work of running, requiring more energy expenditure by the athlete (Baxter, 1993). The fundamental question is whether overpronation is even a pathologic condition that requires treatment. A large study of 1000 runners in whom a variety of lower extremity variables were measured found no relation between pronation and risk of injury (Walter et al., 1989).

Viscoelastic insoles are frequently prescribed to decrease impact loading of the foot during running and jumping and to improve lower extremity kinematics compared with the conventional insoles already present in the athletic shoe. The purported benefits were not demonstrated when critically evaluated in the biomechanical laboratory (Nigg et al., 1988). Therefore although there are individuals who can benefit from orthotic devices over the short term, their widespread use by runners is difficult to support scientifically. Prospective studies are needed to evaluate the efficacy of orthotic devices for treatment and prevention of athletic injuries.

When contemplating prescription of a longitudinal arch support, factors that require consideration include durability, expense, comfort, and effectiveness for treating the pathologic conditions. These devices must be used within a shoe that provides medial, lateral, and dorsal support for the foot. Typically, these inserts are made from a variety of materials, ranging in stiffness from soft to rigid. Softer devices are inexpensive and are constructed of felt, closed-cell foam, or leather and cork (Janisse, 1994; Mann et al., 1981). They are often supplied precut and are distributed "over the counter" in shoe and sporting goods stores. Some trimming to fit the individual shoe may be necessary.

Semirigid supports must be fashioned for the individual foot (Janisse, 1994; Mann et al., 1981). They are made of closed-cell foams of differing densities and rigidity. The materials can be heat-molded to fit the foot. Composite orthoses can be constructed that combine a stiffened underlayer for support with a softer, cushioning layer against the skin. They can be "posted" with greater thickness along the medial side to control pronation. Semirigid orthoses provide the best combination of support and cushioning for runners who require an orthotic device (McKenzie et al., 1985).

Rigid orthoses are made of acrylic from a positive plaster mold (Janisse, 1994; Torg, 1982). A cast of the sole of the foot is made while the foot is in a functional position. The cast is sent to a fabricator, who makes a positive mold from the impression. The acrylic can then be further modified with padding, wedges can be added, or it can be sanded down for a final, "true" fit. These orthoses are the most expensive and are what most athletes know as "orthotics." Because of their rigidity, these devices decrease shock absorption in the heel and can lead to stress injuries in the leg. Extending only to the ball of the foot, they also can adversely affect the forefoot. Interdigital neuromas and sesmoid problems have been associated with their use (Baxter, 1993).

Most longitudinal arch supports should be prescribed for short-term use to treat an identified problem. Once the problem has resolved, it is generally best to remove the support, continuing activity as before. If there is recurrence of the injury, permanent use of the device is indicated. Orthoses used after the original injury has healed may cause secondary problems in the foot.

The UCBL insert is a specialized type of longitudinal arch support designed at the University of California Biomechanics Laboratory (Mann, 1993). This rigid device of fiberglass or polypropylene is custom-molded with the hindfoot in a neutral position. It has walls extending up around the heel that control hindfoot position. The medial wall supports the talonavicular joint, and the lateral wall prevents the forefoot from slipping into abduction. It is used to treat the symptomatic flexible flatfoot.

A HAPAD is a piece of felt with an adhesive backing that is supplied in a variety of thicknesses and sizes. These devices are useful for unweighting specific areas, especially the forefoot. For example, relief of a metatarsal head is achieved by transferring pressure proximally along the shaft, where more area is available to share the load. These devices are inexpensive, readily available from shoe dealers, and the athlete can position the pad himself or herself to obtain the best relief. It is usually best to start with a small size, progressing to larger ones as needed. They are useful for treating a variety of forefoot problems including sesamoiditis, plantar callus, interdigital neuromas, and metatarsalgia.

Several devices can support a single toe and are used to treat hammertoes, metatarsophalangeal (MTP) synovitis, and sprains about the MTP joint. A toe crest has a loop of elastic that is attached to a wedge-shaped piece of felt. The loop passes over the dorsum of the base of the toe, and the wedge fits under the toe. The elastic loop is pulled snug, causing the toe to be bound against the wedge. The toe crest has a small profile and can be worn with most shoes.

A variation on the toe crest has a large, flat cushion to which the elastic strap attaches. It maintains the cushion against the ball of the foot. This device is useful for treating a hammertoe that has accompanying tenderness under the MTP joint. The cushion pad increases the bulk of this orthosis, however, which limits its use to shoewear with an adequate toebox.

Sponge pads are used to spread the toes when treating corns. The sponge is placed distally to keep adjacent toes apart, thereby relieving pressure. They are also used to treat soft corns at the base of a web space. The major disadvantage of these devices is that the lateral toe is forced into abduction. Unless an adequate toebox is available, a corn may develop along the side of the fifth toe.

A variety of orthoses are available for use at the heel. Sponge, felt, and viscoelastic polymer pads can be used to increase cushioning under the heel. Heel cups are cushions with extensions to enclose the sides and back of the heel. The walls of the cup help to contain the normal fat pad of the heel, enhancing its cushioning effect. These are bulkier than simple heel pads and may not fit in all shoes.

Braces

Braces are used for the nonoperative treatment of soft tissue injuries of the ankle and hindfoot. A variety of braces are available, each providing some measure of compression with a stabilizing effect on the ankle. An elastic bandage wrap is used primarily for compression, and when woven in a figure-of-eight pattern around the ankle it provides some stability with limited weight-bearing. It serves as a constant reminder to the patient that an injury is being treated, reinforcing the notion of rest. A variation is the slip-on elastic ankle sleeve. It is a low profile support that acts similarly to an elastic wrap but is easier to wear with a shoe. Another variation is the neoprene sleeve. All of these devices are useful for treating mild injuries or during the final phases of rehabilitation as activities are being advanced.

A stirrup brace supports the ankle with medial and lateral cushioned splints that extend up the distal third of the leg and are connected under the heel by a plastic disc. Velcro straps wrap around the uprights, providing compression and significant stability. These braces allow nearly unrestricted ankle motion while blocking subtalar motion and ankle inversion. They are commonly used for acute treatment of ankle sprains and subtalar injuries.

A lace-up ankle brace is a canvas sleeve with laces running through eylets along the front. Incorporated in the sleeve are rigid bars that, when the sleeve is laced into place, limit ankle inversion. They also limit ankle dorsiflexion and plantarflexion more than the stirrup brace. These braces are useful for treating chronic lateral ankle instability because of their improved durability compared to that of stirrup braces.

An Unna boot is made by wrapping the foot, ankle, and distal leg with a special gauze impregnated with zinc oxide and calamine. This treatment is popular for venous stasis ulcers but has a place in treating acute ankle sprains associated with significant swelling and pain. The "boot" is reserved for the low-level recreational athlete who does not have access to an aggressive rehabilitation program. It provides compression and support for the ankle while permitting weight-bearing. It is used for 1 to 2 weeks, at which time it loosens as swelling resolves.

A removable walking orthosis, or CAM (controlled ankle motion) walker, has many uses for treating injuries of the foot and ankle. It provides stability comparable to a plaster cast with the advantage of being removable, which allows the patient to participate in rehabilitation with motion exercises and allows bathing. A potential disadvantage is that it can be removed by the patient at will and so should not be used on an unreliable patient.

Polypropylene ankle foot orthoses (AFOs) have few indications in the athletic population. They are custom molded, using a Velcro strap to attach them to the leg. AFOs are useful for protecting Achilles tendon reconstructions, for initial nonoperative treatment of peroneal spastic flatfoot (tarsal coalition), and as night splints when treating chronic plantar fasciitis.

Plaster or fiberglass casts provide rigid sta-

bility that is often needed after surgery. Other uses include the treatment of fractures and acute sprains. When applied for an extended period, casts can cause joint stiffness and osteoporosis, so for most athletic injuries the duration of use should be limited. Changing to a removable orthosis is usually feasible by 2 to 3 weeks. Noncompliant patients, however, remain a good indication for prolonged cast immobilization.

Taping Techniques

Taping provides support and compression after acute injuries as well as protection against recurrent injury. Taping is particularly useful forn treating plantar fasciitis and injuries of the longitudinal arch, Achilles tendonitis, and sprains of the ankle and toes. Certain basic principles apply to all taping regimens.

The area to be taped must be clean, dry, and shaved of hair, unless an underwrap is used. An underwrap diminishes the positive grip of the tape on the skin, decreasing the efficiency of the taping. To improve adhesiveness, tincture of benzoin is first applied to the skin. Anchor strips of tape are placed proximally and distally to hold the functional tape in place. Tape should always be applied by overlapping successive strips, as it anchors the tape to the preceding strip and eliminates the chance that a blister will form in an uncovered area between two strips of tape. When applying tape, as with casting, the athlete and physician should both be in comfortable positions.

Tape can loosen with wear, or the edges can unravel, so a covering layer of Coban is added at the end. Some patients have allergies to the adhesive in the tape or to tincture of benzoin, which once identified is avoided thereafter. If not applied properly, blistering or small skin lacerations can result. Tape should be carefully removed with special tape cutters or scissors.

Ankle Taping (Open Basketweave)

The open basketweave technique is useful for acute ankle sprains because it accommodates swelling in the ankle (Bonci, 1982; Cox, 1985). It provides compression but little support. Rolls of 1.0 or 1.5 inch adhesive tape are used with two felt pads each covered on one side with petroleum jelly.

1. The athlete sits on a table with the knee in extension and the lower half of the leg extending past the end of the table. The operator faces the sole of the foot.
2. Felt pads are applied over the dorsum of the ankle and posterior to the heel at the level of the Achilles insertion with the petroleum jelly side against the skin. A proximal anchor strip is placed around three-fourths the circumference of the leg at the midcalf level, leaving the open area in front. Another anchor strip is applied at the level of the metatarsal heads on the ball of the foot, extending on each side onto the dorsum of the foot, leaving the midline free.
3. A vertical stirrup is applied starting at the proximal anchor strip medially, under the heel, and running back up the lateral side of the leg to the anchor strip. This maneuver should pull the ankle under moderate tension into eversion. This first vertical stirrup should be placed as posteriorly as possible.
4. A horizontal stirrup is applied from the distal anchor strip at the medial side of the first metatarsal head, wrapping around the heel, and ending over the anchor strip along the lateral side of the fifth metatarsal head.
5. A second vertical stirrup is applied parallel to the first, overlapping in front of it one-half the width of the tape. Next, a second horizontal stirrup is applied, overlapping the first one in similar fashion, one-half the tape width above it.
6. Vertical and horizontal stirrups are then alternated. Care is taken to leave an anterior opening the entire length of the ankle and foot to allow for swelling. Loose ends can be anchored with longitudinal strips or covered with an elastic bandage or Coban.

Ankle Taping (Figure-of-Eight)

Figure-of-eight taping (Fig. 8.1) provides support for lateral ankle ligaments that are chronically injured (Bonci, 1982). This bandage completely encircles the limb and is therefore not used for an acute injury. Rolls of 1.0 or 1.5 inch adhesive tape are used with two felt pads each covered on one side with petroleum jelly.

1. The athlete sits on a table with the knee in extension and the lower half of the leg extending past the end of the table. The operator faces the sole of the foot.
2. Felt pads are applied over the dorsum of the ankle and posterior to the heel at the level of the Achilles insertion, with the petroleum jelly side against the skin (Fig. 8.1A). After an underwrap is placed, a proximal anchor strip is placed circumferentially around the leg at the midcalf, and a distal one is applied circumferentially around the foot at the level of the distal arch.
3. Heel locks are applied next, using two or three in each direction. The lateral heel lock begins over the lateral distal leg. The tape is run at a 45 degree angle over the front of the distal leg, extending from above the medial malleolus. It then continues in a barberpole configuration inferiorly and posteriorly about the ankle to the lateral side of the heel. It passes under the arch and is brought up to the dorsum of the midfoot. The medial heel lock follows a corkscrew pattern in the opposite direction. It starts on the dorsum of the midfoot and is directed in front of the lateral malleolus, drops inferiorly under the heel, and returns behind the medial malleolus. It then passes posteriorly over the Achilles attachment, wrapping around the lateral side to end on the dorsum of the midfoot (Fig. 8.1B and C).
4. Figure-of-eight strips are then applied using enough tension to place the ankle in slight eversion. The tape starts in front of the medial malleolus and passes down and under the posterior arch to the lateral side. The foot is manually everted at this point. The tape continues up and over the anterior ankle, meeting the starting point, and then continuing posteriorly around the back of the distal leg. It is then directed to the front of the ankle, encircling both

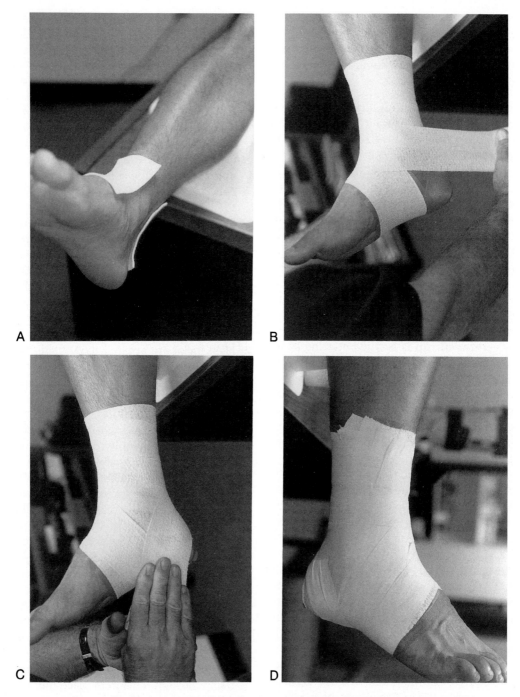

FIGURE 8.1. (A–D) Steps for figure-of-eight ankle taping.

the hindfoot and distal leg. Two to four figure-of-eight wraps are applied.

5. Fill-in strips hold the functional components in place. They should also be applied in an overlapping fashion from distal to proximal (Fig. 8.1D).

Achilles Tendon Taping

Taping is useful for treatment of achilles tendonitis (Bonci, 1982). It restricts dorsiflexion and relieves stress on the tendon. Rolls of 1.0 or 1.5 inch adhesive tape and 2 or

3 inch elastic tape are used with a felt heel pad covered on one side with petroleum jelly.

1. The athlete lies prone on a table with the lower leg extended over the end. The ankle is in a relaxed position of 10 to 15 degrees plantarflexion. The operator stands at the foot of the table.
2. Circumferential anchor strips of adhesive tape are applied proximally at the midcalf and distally just proximal to the metatarsal heads.
3. Longitudinal strips of elastic tape are applied. The first strip starts at the distal anchor under the first metatarsal head, runs to the heel and then the posterolateral leg, ending at the lateral side of the proximal anchor strip. The next strip begins at the distal anchor under the fifth metatarsal head, passes back to the heel, running up the posteromedial leg to end at the medial side of the proximal anchor strip. A third strip is positioned in the midline running from the distal strip along the sole of the foot and then along the posterior calf to end at the anchor strip.
4. Fill-in strips of elastic tape then encircle the foot and leg, beginning distally and overlapping appropriately.

Arch Taping (Low-Dye Technique)

Arch taping is used to treat plantar fasciitis and acute injuries to the longitudinal arch (Fig. 8.2). The technique relieves strain on the plantar fascia and plantar tarsal ligaments (Scranton et al., 1982). One inch adhesive tape is used.

1. The athlete sits or lies supine on a table with the ankle and foot extending over the end. The taper stands at the end of the table.
2. An anchor strip is applied along the metatarsal heads and extends to the dorsum on both medial and lateral sides (Fig. 8.2A).
3. A supportive strip is started under the fifth metatarsal head, crossing under the arch to the medial heel and then wrapping posteriorly around the heel just below the

Achilles tendon (Fig. 8.2B). It is continued down the lateral side of the heel to the sole, where it crosses itself under the arch before ending under the first metatarsal head (Fig. 8.2C). A second strip of tape is placed similarly.
4. Three fill-ins are placed over the anchor strips at the metatarsal head level, sandwiching the ends of the supportive strips and locking them in place. Additional fill-ins are used on the plantar aspect of the foot (Fig. 8.2D), or the foot is encircled with Coban.

Great Toe Taping

Great-toe taping is used to treat turf toe (Fig. 8.3) and sesamoid injuries to support the great toe and limit dorsiflexion (Sammarco, 1993). One inch adhesive tape is used.

1. The athlete sits on a table with the knee extended and the heel at the edge of the table.
2. An anchor is placed circumferentially around the toe and about the forefoot at the metatarsal head level (Fig. 8.3A).
3. Figure-of-eight supports are then applied. The strips are started under the first metatarsal head from the anchor, run along the medial side of the toe, and pass over the dorsum of the toe proximal to the interphalangeal joint (Fig. 8.3B). The tape is then routed from the base of the metatarsal, crossing laterally over the toe to end at the distal anchor. This procedure is repeated two or three times.
4. Fill-in strips are then placed from distal to proximal to lock the supportive strips to the anchors (Fig. 8.3C).

Buddy Taping

Buddy taping is used to treat fractures and dislocations of the lesser toes. The adjacent normal toe acts as a splint for the injured one. One-half inch adhesive tape is used. A small wisp of cotton, felt, or lamb's wool is inserted between the toes. The tape is then wrapped circumferentially about the two toes at least twice.

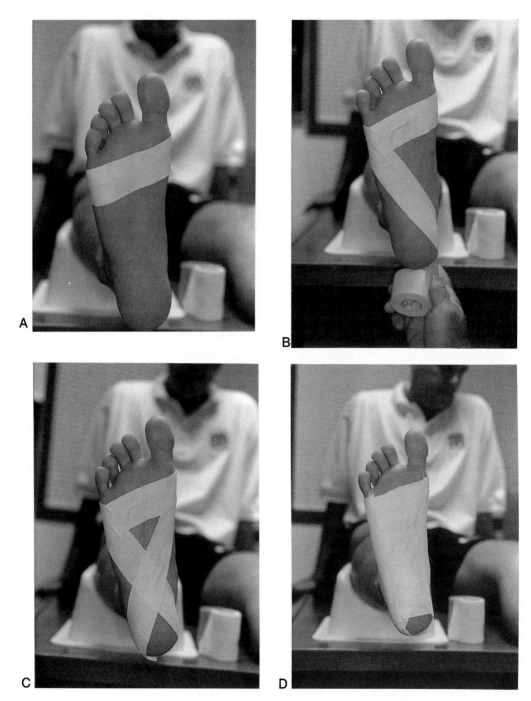

FIGURE 8.2. (A–D) Steps for plantar fascia taping.

Injection Techniques

Injections are useful for diagnosing and treating a variety of foot and ankle disorders. Diagnostic injections are performed with local anesthetic and are placed in a joint, tendon sheath, or specific area of tenderness. The athlete is then asked to perform activities that would normally cause pain to confirm the diagnosis.

In the forefoot, for example, injections are used to differentiate an interdigital neuroma

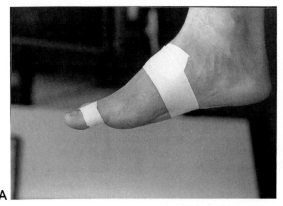
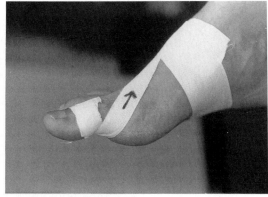

A   B

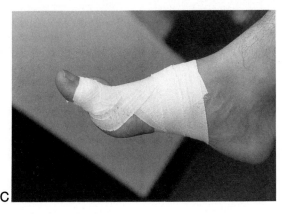

C

FIGURE 8.3. (A–C) Steps for turf toe taping.

from metatarsophalangeal (MTP) joint syno-vitis. Often an injection can discriminate ankle from subtalar joint pain or ankle from-peroneal tendon pain. Once the site of pain has been identified, appropriate treatment can be administered. Steroid injections are indicated for a number of conditions. Ste-roids, however, are *contraindicated* near the Achilles or posterior tibial tendons.

Diagnostic Local Anesthetic Injection

The athlete is first questioned about any known allergies to local anesthetics.

1. A mixture of 1% lidocaine and 0.5% bupi-vacaine (Marcaine) provides a block lasting 4 to 5 hours. Solutions with epinephrine are not used. The local anesthetics are drawn into a single syringe. For most forefoot injections a 3 ml syringe provides an adequate volume, whereas for most hindfoot and ankle injections a 5 ml syringe is used. For most injections in the foot and ankle, a 25 gauge 1.5 inch needle is selected.

2. The area to be injected is identified and the overlying skin prepared with an antiseptic solution. A topical anesthetic such as ethyl chloride is sprayed on the skin at the injection site. The needle is then placed through the skin into the area of pathol-ogy. It is important that minimal or no local anesthetic is injected in the skin or surrounding tissue. The anesthetics are preferentially injected in the area of sus-pected pathology. This caution ensures that only the chosen area is blocked, en-hancing the usefulness of this test for determining the source of pain.

Steroid Injection

Injection of corticosteroid is performed in a manner similar to that for a simple local anesthetic injection.

1. A syringe with local anesthetic is prepared
as above. A second 3 ml syringe is filled
with 1 ml of triamcinolone or dexame-
thasone if a water soluble steroid is preferred. The skin is prepared with an antiseptic solution, and a topical anesthetic is
applied.
2. The local anesthetic is injected and the
needle advanced to the apppropriate position. The needle is left in place; the syringe
is then detached and replaced with the
syringe containing the steroid. The steroid
is injected, usually a volume of 0.3 to 0.5
ml for the forefoot joints and interdigital
neuromas and 1 ml in the hindfoot joints
or in the plantar fascia attachment.
3. The needle is again left in place, and the
steroid-containing syringe is removed and
replaced with the local anesthetic syringe.
The needle is then slowly withdrawn with
only local anesthetic injected. This step
ensures that no steroid is inadvertently
left in the subcutaneous tissue or skin.

References

American Academy of Orthopaedic Surgeons:
Taping, bandaging, orthotics. In: American
Academy of Orthopaedic Surgeons, Athletic
Training and Sports Medicine, 2nd ed, pp
647–704, Rosemont, IL, AAOS, 1991

Andreasson G, Lindenberger U, Renstrom P, Peterson L: Torque developed at simulated
sliding between sports shoes and an artificial
turf. Am J Sports Med 14:225–230, 1986

Baxter DE: The foot in running. In: Mann RA,
Coughlin MJ (eds): Surgery of the Foot
and Ankle, pp 1225–1239, St. Louis, Mosby,
1993

Bonci C: Adhesive strapping techniques. Clin
Sports Med 1:99–116, 1982

Cook SD, Kester MA, Brunet ME, Haddad RJ:
Biomechanics of running shoe performance.
Clin Sports Med 4:619–626, 1985

Cox J: Surgical and nonsurgical treatment of acute
ankle sprains. Clin Orthop 198:118–126, 1985

Janisse DJ: Indications and prescriptions for orthoses in sports. Orthop Clin North Am
25:95–107, 1994

Lutter LD: Foot-related knee problems in the long
distance runner. Foot Ankle 1:112–116, 1980

Mann RA: Conservative treatment of the foot. In
Mann RA, Coughlin MJ (eds): Surgery of the
Foot and Ankle, pp 141–149, St. Louis, Mosby,
1993

Mann RA, Baxter DE, Lutter LD: Running sympo-
sium. Foot Ankle 1:190–224, 1981

McKenzie DC, Clement DB, Taunton JE: Running
shoes, orthotics, and injuries. Sports Med
2:334–347, 1985

Nigg BM, Herzog W, Read LJ: Effect of viscoelastic
shoe insoles on vertical impact forces in heel-
toe running. Am J Sports Med 16:70–76, 1988

Sammarco GJ: Turf toe. AAOS Instructional
Course Lect 42:207–212, 1993

Scranton PE, Pedegana LR, Whitesl JP: Gait analysis alterations in support phase forces using
supportive devices. Am J Sports Med 10:6–11,
1982

Torg JS: Athletic footwear and orthotic appliances.
Clin Sports Med 1:157–175, 1982

Index